HDP

HYDROXYP
    DIPH(

D1433513

MDP

METHYLENE
    DIPHOSPHONATE

CLINICIAN'S GUIDE TO NUCLEAR MEDICINE

BENIGN AND MALIGNANT BONE DISEASE

Clinician's Guide to Nuclear Medicine

Benign and Malignant Bone Disease

J H McKillop
Muirhead Professor of Medicine
Royal Infirmary
Glasgow, UK

I Fogelman
Consultant Physician
Department of Nuclear Medicine
Guy's Hospital
London, UK

CHURCHILL LIVINGSTONE
EDINBURGH • LONDON • MELBOURNE • NEW YORK 1991

CHURCHILL LIVINGSTONE
Medical Division of Longman Group UK Limited

Distributed in the United States of America by
Churchill Livingstone Inc., 1560 Broadway, New York,
N.Y. 10036, and by associated companies, branches
and representatives throughout the world.

First published 1991

ISBN 0-443-04436-8

British Library Cataloguing in Publication Data
McKillop, James H.
  Benign and malignant bone disease.
  1. Man. Bones. Tumours. Diagnosis. Magnetic resonance
  imaging
  I. Title II. Fogelman, Ignac III. Series
  616. 992710757

Library of Congress Cataloging in Publication Data
McKillop, James H.
  Clinician's guide to nuclear medicine: benign and malignant
  bone disease/J.H. McKillop, I. Fogelman.
      p. cm.
  Includes index.
  ISBN 0-443-04436-8
  1. Bones — Radionuclide imaging. I. Fogelman, Ignac, 1948–
  II. Title.
  [DNLM: 1. Bone and Bones — radionuclide imaging.
  WE 200 M478c]
  RC930.5.M38 1990
  616.7'107575 — dc20
  DNLM/DLC   90–15016
  for Library of Congress   CIP

Produced by Longman Singapore Publishers Pte Ltd
Printed in Singapore

Preface

Nuclear medicine has an established place in modern medicine. The specialty is now almost 50 years old, the first clinically useful applications of the radioactive tracer method being developed in the late 1940s and early 1950s.

The scope of nuclear medicine has grown spectacularly in this period, but its nature has also altered due to the introduction and development of other imaging modalities, notably X-ray CT scanning, magnetic resonance imaging and diagnostic ultrasound. Nuclear medicine, however, remains unique in its ability to yield functionally based rather than anatomically based information.

This series of books entitled 'A Clinician's Guide to Nuclear Medicine' intends to present the clinical utility of Nuclear Medicine to all doctors, whether in general medicine/surgery or specialized disciplines, i.e. Neurology and Psychiatry, Gastroenterology, Cancer, Cardiology, Nephrourology etc.

Under the auspices of the British Nuclear Medicine Society, expert physicians from the United Kingdom have been asked to write these books. As the title of the series implies, the book should act as a guide to clinicians interested in the radioactive tracer method in their own specialty or in clinical practice. In general a series Editor has co-ordinated this development, Amersham International plc has helped to sponsor the publication of these books, and Churchill Livingstone has been appointed as Publisher for this series.

The British Nuclear Medicine Society hopes that these books will help the clinician to understand the potential and wide-ranging applications of the radioactive tracer method to Medicine in general and to clinical problem-solving in particular.

The books are well illustrated, have been purposely

designed as handbooks, and contain many useful tables and diagrams. The discussion of clinical case material is included, wherever relevant.

London, 1991   P. J. Ell

Contents

1 | Radionuclide Bone Scanning

Bone imaging using a radionuclide was first reported by Fleming and his colleagues in 1961. They found that the tracer strontium-85 (^{85}Sr) localized preferentially in areas of osteoblastic activity compared to normal bone and that a scan could be used as an index of bone repair. They concluded that scanning bone lesions was both practical

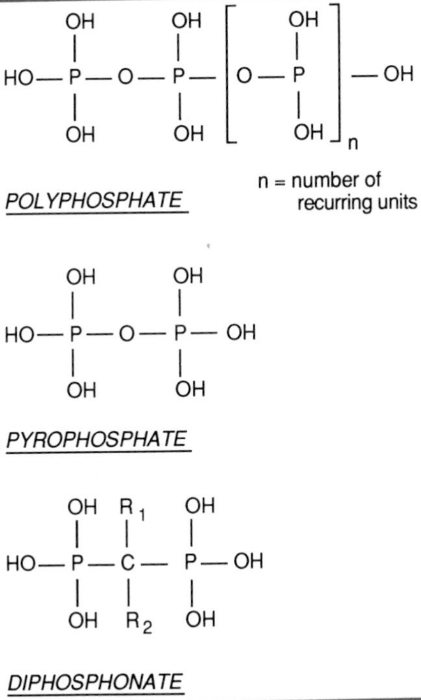

Fig. 1.1 **Chemical formulae of bone scan agents. The groups R_1 and R_2 differ in the various diphosphonates.**

and informative. Various other skeletal imaging agents, notably strontium-87 and fluorine-18, were introduced in the 1960s and by 1970 bone scanning had become a clinically acceptable procedure in patients with malignant disease. The radiopharmaceuticals available at that time all had shortcomings in either their physical characteristics or physiological properties, thus limiting use of the technique. The situation was changed dramatically in 1971 when Subramanian and McAfee described the first of the technetium-99m-labelled phosphate compounds.

The initial ^{99m}Tc phosphate was a polyphosphate (Fig. 1.1). This showed good skeletal uptake with relatively low background (non-skeletal) uptake. The ability to label with ^{99m}Tc, which has near ideal physical characteristics for use with the gamma camera, was another major factor in improving the quality of images compared to previous bone-seeking radiopharmaceuticals. Technetium-99m pyrosphosphate (Fig. 1.1) showed improved bone-to-background activity ratios compared to polyphosphate. A third group of compounds – the diphosphonates (Fig. 1.1) – had the advantage over the polyphosphates and pyrophosphates of resisting breakdown in vivo by tissue phosphatases. Studies with ^{99m}Tc-diphosphonates for bone scanning rapidly demonstrated improved image quality compared to previously available compounds. Since then various diphosphonates with differing physiological properties have been introduced. The ^{99m}Tc-diphosphonates have become established as the bone scan agents of choice and have replaced the polyphosphates and pyrophosphates in clinical practice. The diphosphonate most widely used for bone scanning at present is ^{99m}Tc-methylene diphosphonate (^{99m}Tc-MDP).

MECHANISM OF SKELETAL UPTAKE OF THE DIPHOSPHONATE

Following intravenous administration the diphosphonates show fairly rapid blood clearance with less than 10% of the injected activity of ^{99m}Tc-MDP remaining in the blood pool 1 hour post injection and less than 2% at 4 hours. Clearance occurs principally by a combination of skeletal uptake and urinary excretion. The proportions of radiopharmaceutical bound to the skeleton and that excreted by the urinary tract vary for different diphosphonates.

Skeletal blood flow influences local uptake of diphosphonates – avascular areas of bone will show absence of uptake, while areas of high vascularity show increased uptake. Various animal models, however, have shown that vascularity alone does not explain skeletal uptake of diphosphonates and the uptake of diphosphonate in bone lesions will be increased to a greater extent than that of labelled microspheres which simply reflect blood flow. The crucial influence on diphosphonate uptake appears to be osteoblastic activity, with areas of high osteoblastic activity demonstrating high diphosphonate uptake. Diphosphonate accumulating in bone appears to do so on the bone surface with tracer being incorporated into the complex bone mineral crystal hydroxyapatite rather than into the collagenous matrix. Because of the binding to bone surfaces and the resistance to breakdown by tissue phosphatases, bone uptake of diphosphonates is long lasting, and there is certainly no significant loss of the radiopharmaceutical from bone over the time span of a bone scan.

The basis of use of the bone scan in clinical practice is that virtually all lesions within the skeleton will excite a local osteoblastic response and an increase in vascularity. It should be noted that this response is non-specific and occurs in a wide variety of pathologies such as trauma, infection, malignancy etc. The osteoblastic response and increased vascularity will result in a local accumulation of tracer and will be seen on the bone scan as a 'hot spot'.

Some degree of osteoblastic response is usually present even in lesions which appear osteolytic when bone metastases are X-rayed, so that in this situation a hot spot will be seen on the scan. There are some exceptions to this general rule of which myelomatosis is the most common example. Because of the lack of osteoblastic response in myeloma, the bone scan often fails to show hot spots at established lesions. In the case of a large, purely osteolytic lesion, whether from myeloma or from other causes, an area of decreased uptake (photopenia) may be seen on the bone scan.

Radionuclide bone scanning: Bone scan or bone X-ray?

It is relevant to consider the properties which we require in a bone scanning agent. MDP is characterized by a higher bone uptake and, hence, better bone-to-soft tissue ratio than earlier diphosphonates. This provides good quality skeletal images with clearly recognizable detail of the skeleton. More important, however, in lesion detection is the lesion-to-normal bone uptake ratio. Agents which show high uptake in normal bone could theoretically make lesion detection more difficult. A number of diphosphonates which show lower normal bone uptake and higher lesion-to-normal bone ratios are currently being investigated, though they have not as yet been shown to have any significant advantage over MDP in practice.

BONE SCAN OR BONE X-RAY?

Changes on bone X-rays reflect alterations in bone structure. This may occur due to disruption of bone integrity, as in a fracture, or due to changes in bone mineral content. Bone mineral content results from a balance between bone resorption or destruction and bone repair. Bone destruction is usually mediated via osteoclasts while bone repair is the function of osteoblasts. Alterations in bone mineral density can produce bone X-ray abnormalities. If bone destruction predominates, the appearance will be of decreased density – radiolucencies or osteolytic lesions – while bone repair produces areas of increased density – radiodensities or sclerotic lesions. Both of these processes can be seen in metastatic disease.

It has long been recognized that bone X-rays are relatively insensitive in detecting skeletal metastases. This problem arises because of the considerable structural changes required before any lesion visible on X-ray occurs and it has been shown that a lesion in a trabecular bone must be greater than 1–1.5 cm in diameter with a loss of around 50% of bone mineral before radiolucencies will be seen on a standard bone X-ray. Similarly, early on in repair insufficient mineral has been laid down to produce radiodensities.

The radionuclide bone scan is dependent on a completely different principle. As discussed above the major factor controlling deposition of bone-seeking radiophar-maceuticals in the skeleton is osteoblastic activity. The bone scan thus gives a pictorial representation of bone function rather than structure. Most pathologies affecting bone will excite an attempt at bone repair by the osteoblasts and thus be associated with locally increased uptake of the bone agent, with a resultant hot spot on the scan. This functional change in bone often occurs in the disease process at an earlier stage than structural changes detectable on bone X-ray. For this reason the bone scan is normally much more sensitive than radiography in detecting skeletal pathologies. However, the osteoblastic response is common to many pathologies and the bone scan changes are accordingly non-specific. For this reason bone scan abnormalities are often correlated with other investigations, notably local X-rays, to determine their aetiology.

The bone X-ray and bone scan are thus complementary. Because of its greater specificity the bone X-ray should be employed first when there is a localized problem likely to be associated with marked changes in bone structure. A fracture is a good example of this situation. The bone X-ray should also be used to detect pathologies which do not typically excite an osteoblastic response, myeloma being the most common example. In a patient with localized bone pain but negative X-rays a bone scan, with its increased sensitivity, is often useful in detecting early pathology. This approach is valuable in patients with suspected bone infection (see Chapter 3). The bone scan should also be the initial investigation when looking for disseminated disease, such as metastases, firstly because of its ability to pick up earlier lesions, and secondly because a whole-body survey can be obtained at a much lower radiation dose. The bone scan provides excellent visualization of the whole skeleton and is of great value in assessing areas which are radiographically difficult such as the ribs, sternum and scapulae.

The precise inter-relationship between bone X-rays and bone scans in different pathologies will be considered in the following chapters, but the respective advantages of each are listed in Table 1.1.

Table 1.1 **Comparison of bone X-ray and bone scintigraphy**

Advantages of bone X-ray
Easily obtained **High specificity** **Positive in purely osteolytic processes**

Advantages of bone scintigraphy
High sensitivity **Ease of whole-body studies** **Assessment of radiologically difficult areas**

PERFORMING A BONE SCAN

Methylene diphosphonate is supplied in a vial which contains sufficient material for several patients. Labelling is a simple procedure. Technetium-99m pertechnetate, freshly prepared from a generator, is added to the vial at room temperature and the vial gently swirled until the powder is completely dissolved. The resultant solution is clear or slightly opalescent and colourless. The Administration of Radioactive Substances Advisory Committee (ARSAC) maximum recommended dose for bone scanning of adults is 600 MBq (16.2 mCi) though activities of up to 25 mCi are used in other countries. The radiopharmaceutical is given as a slow intravenous injection over 30 seconds.

With methylene diphosphonate a minimum of 2 hours should elapse between injection and imaging, but better quality studies will be obtained by waiting for 3 or 4 hours when background soft tissue activity is further reduced. A longer delay between injection and imaging is especially important when bone uptake is likely to be poor, eg in osteoporosis or when high soft tissue uptake is present, eg in grossly obese patients. In the period between injection and imaging the patient should be encouraged to drink at least 1.5 – 2 litres of fluid unless there is a clear contraindication to this, such as oliguric renal failure or severe cardiac failure. High fluid intake encourages increased renal filtration and may increase the rate of clearance of unbound (soft tissue) activity thus increasing the contrast between bone to soft tissues. More importantly, the high urine output reduces the radiation dose incurred by the bladder, the critical organ in bone scanning, firstly by increasing the urine volume in the bladder thus diluting the activity per unit volume of urine and secondly by encouraging frequent voiding.

Bone scanning can be performed using a rectilinear scanner, but in modern practice a gamma camera should be used. The photopeak of the camera should be set on 140 keV. A low energy all purpose parallel hole (LEAP) or a high resolution collimator is employed. Whole-body bone scans may be performed using the camera in the scanning mode but this is associated with poorer resolution than the alternative of multiple spot views (Fig. 1.2 A, B, C). Therefore, provided a wide field of view camera is available, multiple spot views is the preferred technique. Images can be recorded directly onto film from the camera oscilloscope (analogue images) but storing of data on computer and subsequent imaging (digital images) is preferable as it allows image processing if necessary and ensures correct photographic exposure each time. The precise technique for acquiring spot views varies in different departments but typically views of the axial skeleton will contain 500–750K counts, with limb views being acquired for a fixed time such as 180 seconds.

There is some debate about what constitutes an adequate bone scan study in a routine patient. Even in patients with known malignancy, in many departments only the skull and axial skeleton (including pelvis) are imaged unless the patient has symptoms in the limbs. In others, the limbs are routinely imaged. This increases the time taken for a bone scan from around 25–30 minutes up to 40–45 minutes. The yield of limb views in asymptomatic patients is small but in view of the importance of not missing metastases in the shaft of long bones the ideal of obtaining limb views in all patients should be followed whenever possible.

Certain modifications to the standard bone scan technique may be required in particular circumstances. When looking for osteomyelitis, or occasionally for vascular tumours, a three phase bone scan is obtained. The area of the skeleton for study is placed under the gamma camera

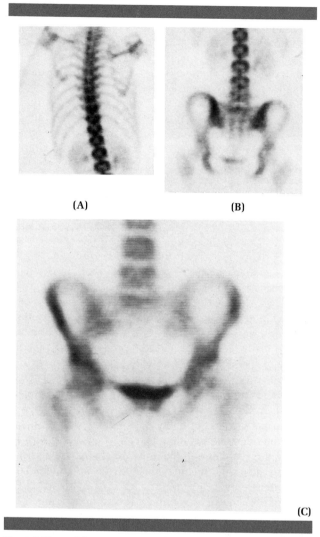

(A)

(B)

(C)

Fig. 1.2 **Normal bone scan – overlapping spot views of the thoracic spine (A), the lumbar spine and posterior pelvis (B), and the anterior pelvis (C).**

and the tracer is injected as a bolus. Dynamic images are obtained every 1–2 seconds for the first 60 seconds to demonstrate perfusion (Phase 1). At 5 minutes post injection a 60-second image is obtained of the blood pool (Phase 2). Standard delayed static images are obtained at 4 hours (Phase 3). A normal three phase bone scan is shown in Fig. 1.3 A, B, C. Three phase bone scans are of value in differentiating cellulitis from osteomyelitis (see Chapter 3).

Special techniques are required on occasions to differentiate bony lesions of the pelvis from urinary activity. A full bladder may obscure considerable detail of the bony pelvis because of the radioactive urine contained in it (Fig. 1.4). Patients should be asked to empty their bladder immediately before the pelvic views are obtained. If doubts remain as to whether activity lies within the bladder or pelvic bones, then squat views should be obtained, with the patient squatting above the gamma camera. Such images usually separate bony and urinary bladder activity (Fig. 1.5 A, B). If doubt still persists then 24-hour post-injection images may be helpful – by this time all soft tissue and urinary activity should have cleared and any residual activity is likely to be bony. Twenty-four hour images are rarely necessary but can also occasionally be useful in making clearer lesions that are equivocal on 4-hour images.

An additional technique which may be useful in defining areas of skeletal abnormality more precisely is single photon emission computed tomography (SPECT). Labelled diphosphonate is injected as usual and images of the region of interest are obtained at multiple projections (usually 36) over a 180° or 360° arc by rotating the gamma camera around the patient. The computer is then used to construct tomographic slices from the multiple planar views. This method is especially valuable when detailed anatomical localization is required, eg within a vertebral body, (Fig. 1.6 A, B, C) or when cold lesions are being sought.

The normal bone scan
The main characteristic of the bone scan is that corresponding structures on the right and left of the body show equivalent activity, that is, there is symmetry about the midline. Areas of greater bone mass, eg the pelvis will show greater activity than thinner areas such as the forearm bones. There is also increased uptake at sites of stress

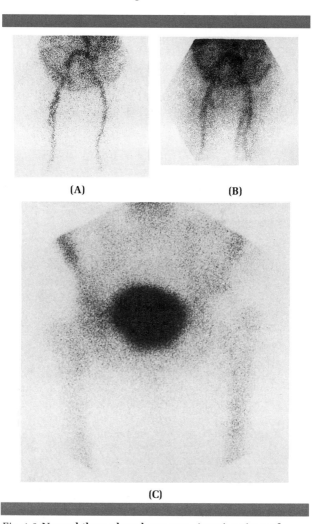

(A)   (B)

(C)

Fig. 1.3 **Normal three phase bone scan. Anterior views of pelvis and hips from 63-year-old male with previous left total hip replacement. No discrete focus of increased activity is seen on the perfusion (A), or blood pool images (B), though intravascular activity is clearly seen. On the delayed image (C),a photon deficient area is seen, representing the hip replacement, but no increased tracer accumulation is seen in association with the prosthesis.**

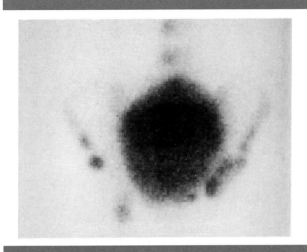

Fig. 1.4 Anterior view of pelvis in patient with disseminated breast cancer. Some focal hot spots are seen in the spine, pelvis and right femur but much of the pelvis is obscured by the distended bladder.

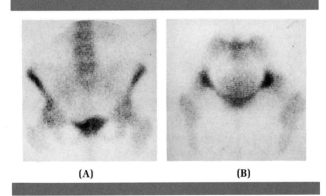

(A)   (B)

Fig. 1.5 (A) Anterior view of pelvis shows increased activity over the pubis. It is unclear if this is due to bony pathology or urinary bladder activity. The squat view (B) demonstrates that the pubis is normal.

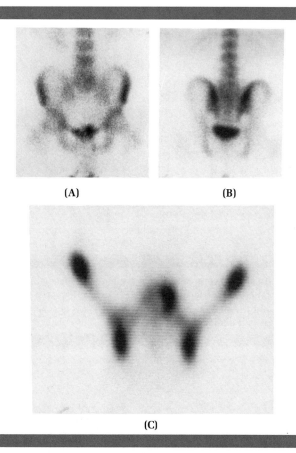

(A)   (B)

(C)

Fig. 1.6 **39-year-old woman with low back pain and a possible sclerotic lesion in L5 on X-ray. Planar anterior (A) and posterior (B) bone scans appear normal. The SPECT image (C) shows clear assymetry of uptake in the body of L5 confirming the presence of a lesion.**

such as periarticular areas or areas of large muscle insertions.

The vault of the skull shows a relatively low count rate. Some uptake may be seen in the regions of the sutures, even in adults. The base of the skull shows relatively higher uptake, and more focally increased uptake in the sphenoid is a not infrequent normal finding. Though not normal variants, it should be realized that frontal sinusitis (Fig. 1.7) or dental disease (Fig. 1.8) are commonly present and may cause a reaction in adjacent bone to produce a hot spot on the bone scan. Hyperostosis frontalis also causes increased uptake on the bone scan (Fig. 1.9 A, B, C).

In the cervical spine vertebrae are relatively small and lie closely. Thus, individual vertebrae may not be visible without the use of ultra-high resolution collimators. Uptake in the anterior neck is usually due to the thyroid cartilage. If there is a radiopharmaceutical problem, uptake of free ^{99m}Tc by the thyroid may produce a similar appearance, but this is usually detectable from the classical thyroid shape and by the uptake of the free ^{99m}Tc by the stomach. Because of the reliability of modern bone scanning agents such problems are rare.

In the thorax the sternum is usually clearly distinguished and focally increased uptake is common in the sternoclav-

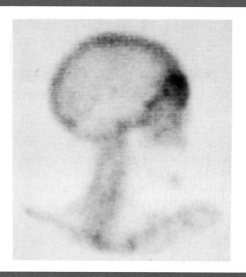

Fig. 1.7 **Right lateral view of skull demonstrating increased uptake in the frontal bone due to frontal sinusitis.**

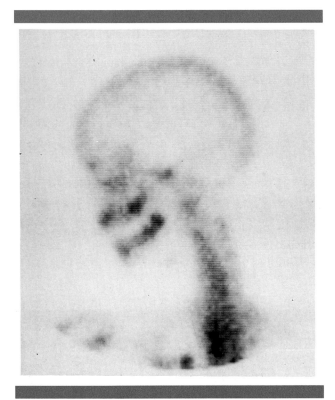

Fig. 1.8 **Extensive caries with increased uptake in the maxilla and mandible.**

icular and sternomanubrial joints. The individual ribs are clearly seen on the anterior and posterior projections. The posterior ribs may show a stippled appearance. This is thought to be due to muscle insertions pulling on the bone and creating locally increased bone turnover. The scapulae are well seen and show high uptake in the angles, again due to muscle stresses. It may be difficult sometimes to distinguish scapular and rib lesions. This problem can be resolved by asking the patient to abduct the arm and repeating the image – scapular lesions will move, rib lesions will not.

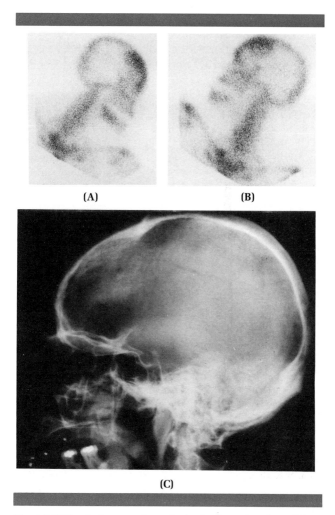

(A)   (B)

(C)

Fig. 1.9 **Diffusely increased uptake in the frontal region of the skull (A and B) characteristic of hyperostosis frontalis, which is confirmed on X-ray (C).**

In the upper thoracic spine the intervertebral spaces often cannot be resolved, but this is usually possible in the lower thoracic and lumbar spine. The spinous processes and transverse processes are also often visible in the lower thoracic and lumbar spine.

The presence of urinary activity in the bladder has already been mentioned. Variations in bladder shape, bladder diverticula or bladder displacement by pelvic tumours may complicate the re-cognition of the nature of this activity. In the posterior pelvic view the sacro-iliac joints are areas of normally high uptake.

The uptake in the shafts of the long bones is relatively low, with more activity being seen in their ends. Increased activity around the patellae is common and of no particular significance (Fig. 1.10). Muscle insertions may cause areas of increased uptake, notably at the deltoid tuberosity in the humerus. In the hands and feet details of individual carpal or tarsal bones cannot usually be made out using the standard collimator but the metacarpals, metatarsals and the phalanges are easily visible (Fig. 1.11). More detail can be seen if a high resolution collimator and a prolonged acquisition time are used (Fig. 1.12).

Safety of bone scanning

As with all radionuclide tests the safety of bone scanning must be considered separately for radiation exposure and adverse drug reactions. For the ARSAC adult recommended maximum injected activity of 600 MBq the estimated whole body radiation dose is 5 mSv. The critical organ is the bladder. As discussed above the radiation dose to the bladder is minimized by having the patient drink large volumes of fluid and voiding urine frequently following injection. The radiation dose from a bone scan is substantially less than from a radiographic skeletal survey.

The diphosphonates are now the radiopharmaceuticals most commonly reported to cause adverse reactions, though in absolute terms the numbers are still extremely small – less than 10 per year in the UK. The symptoms are typical of hypersensitivity reactions. They are usually mild, consisting of mild urticaria, but collapse and full blown anaphylaxis may also occur. Normally, apart from explanation and reassurance, antihistamines or no treatment at all are required but rarely more severe reactions may require full resuscitation and administration of corticosteroids.

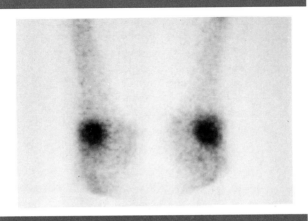

Fig. 1.10 **Increased uptake in both patellae. This may be a normal variant and occur in the absence of pathology (as in this patient).**

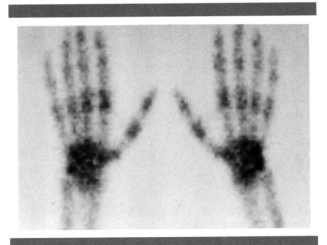

Fig. 1.11 **Images of hands, using standard collimator. Individual metacarpals and phalanges can be seen but no detail of the carpal bones or the small joints of the hands is visible.**

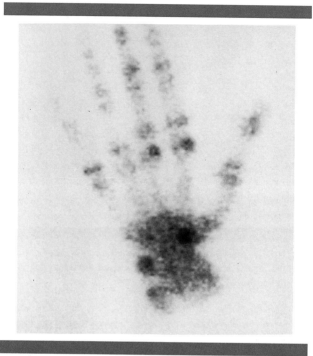

Fig. 1.12 **Image of hand acquired for 15 minutes, using a high resolution collimator. More detail of the joints is visible compared to Fig. 1.11. Several hot spots due to degenerative disease are seen.**

Diphosphonate administration should not be repeated in a patient with a past history of reaction to them.

In summary, the radiation and hypersensitivity risks associated with bone scanning are sufficiently low to make the technique widely applicable in clinical practice.

SOFT TISSUE UPTAKE OF BONE SCAN AGENTS

Soft tissue uptake of the diphosphonate bone scan agents can be of value in identifying unsuspected extraskeletal abnormalities. It is also important as a potential source of confusion in interpreting the bone scan. The causes of abnormal non-skeletal diphosphonate uptake can conveniently be divided into those in the urinary tract and those elsewhere in the body.

The urinary tract is the route of excretion for tracer which has not bound to the skeleton and renal images can be seen on normal bone scans. The renal images should be inspected for asymmetry or for absence of one kidney (Fig. 1.13) which may be due to previous removal or to non-function. Before concluding that a kidney is absent it is essential to ensure that the patient does not merely have a low-lying kidney, which may be visible only on the anterior pelvic views rather than the lumbar spine views. Space-occupying lesions within the kidney may also be detected on the bone scan (Fig. 1.14) but the sensitivity for this is low. Renal tract obstruction may also be first identified on a bone scan. Minor degrees of calyceal retention (Fig. 1.15) are not significant, but evidence of hydronephrosis

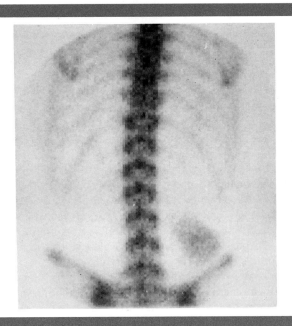

Fig. 1.13 **Posterior view of lower thoracic and lumbar spine. The right kidney is clearly seen but the left renal image is absent due to unsuspected non-function of this kidney.**

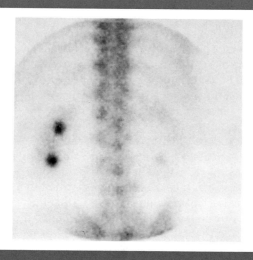

Fig. 1.14 **Posterior view of lower thoracic and lumbar spine. The right kidney shows a large cold area due to space-occupying lesion. Subsequent investigation showed this to be a previously unsuspected renal carcinoma. The left kidney shows calyceal pooling of urine.**

(Fig. 1.16) should always be reported as this may be the first indication of the abnormality. In the case of pelvic tumours obstructing the lower urinary tract, hydroureter may also be picked up on the bone scan (Fig. 1.17 A, B).

Problems caused by residual urine in the bladder or by abnormalities of bladder shape have already been discussed. Difficulties may also arise if a patient is incontinent of urine – spots of radioactivity deposited on the skin may mimic metastases in the underlying bone.

Non-urinary tract uptake of the bone agents may arise from many causes. Tissue infarction is an important group. The mechanism of uptake in this situation is not entirely clear but may be related to desposition of calcium within necrotic tissue (microcalcification). Bone agent uptake may be seen in cerebral infarction or in myocardial infarction (Fig. 1.18 A, B). Indeed, bone scan agents, particularly

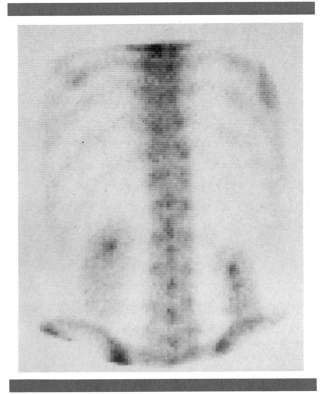

Fig. 1.15 **Posterior view of lower thoracic and lumbar spine.
Upper pole calyceal pooling of urine is seen in both kidneys.
This is of no clinical significance.**

^{99m}Tc-pyrophosphate, have been used as hot spot imaging
agents for diagnosis of myocardial infarction. Skeleton
muscle necrosis, either due to myositis or trauma may lead
to uptake of the bone scanning agents (Fig. 1.19). In patients with sickle cell disease, repeated episodes of splenic
infarction may result in massive uptake of the bone scanning agent (Fig. 1.20). A recent surgical scar may also show
as a hot spot on the bone scan (Fig. 1.21).

Soft tissue calcification may also cause bone scan abnormalities which may be either local, as in calcinosis circumscripta (Fig. 1.22), vascular calcification (Fig. 1.23 A,

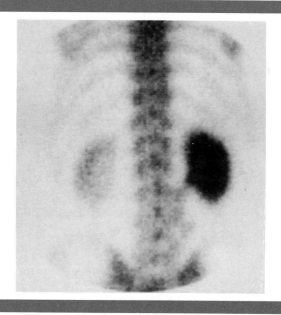

Fig. 1.16 **Posterior view of thoracic spine and lumbar spine from 48-year-old man with back pain. No bony abnormalities are seen but there is a clinically unsuspected right hydronephrosis with early hydroureter.**

B) and costal cartilage calcification (Fig. 1.24) or more gen-eralized as in hypercalcaemia (Fig. 1.25). Amyloidosis is a further condition which may cause diffuse uptake of tracer in the affected organs (Fig. 1.26).

Breast uptake of bone agents is often seen incidentally and when symmetrical is a normal finding (Fig. 1.27). Asymmetrical or unilateral breast uptake is of more impor-tance and merits investigation for possible breast carci-noma.

Metastatic disease is another cause of abnormal bone scan agent uptake. Hepatic metastases may on occasions produce local uptake of the diphosphonates (Fig. 1.28 A, B). This is most often seen with secondaries from colonic cancer but may occur with other primaries. Lung metasta-

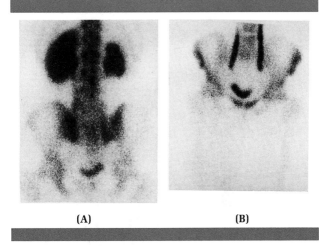

Fig. 1.17 **(A) Posterior view of lumbar spine from 32-year-old woman with locally recurrent carcinoma of uterine cervix, demonstrating bilateral hydronephrosis. The anterior view of pelvis (B) demonstrates bilateral hydroureter.**

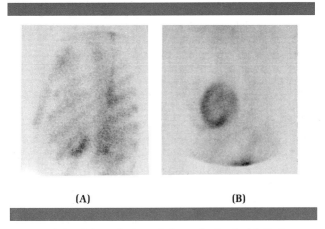

Fig. 1.18 **(A) Left lateral view of chest, obtained with ^{99m}Tc-pyrophosphate, demonstrating uptake within a posterior myocardial infarction. (B) Left lateral view of a resting myocardial perfusion study in the same patient using ^{99m}Tc-MIBI shows a corresponding area of hypoperfusion.**

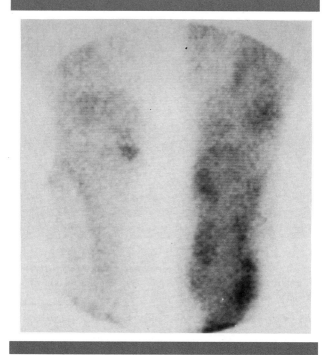

Fig. 1.19 **Anterior view of knees from patient with extensive crush injuries to left leg. Marked uptake is seen in the muscles of the thigh and upper calf, reflecting extensive muscle necrosis.**

ses, notably from osteosarcoma, may also cause abnormalities on the bone scan. This, however, is too variable to be of value as a screening test for lung metastases. Soft tissue metastases at other sites may also show bone agent uptake occasionally (see Fig. 2.16 page 50).

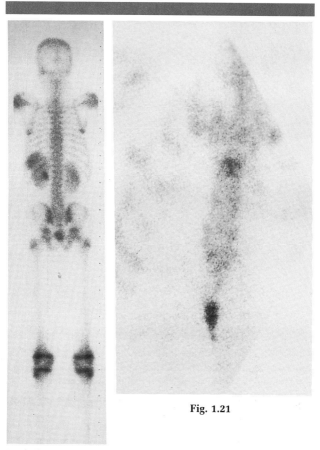

Fig. 1.21

Fig. 1.20

Fig. 1.20 **Whole-body bone scan from an 18-year-old male with sickle cell disease (posterior view). There is marked uptake in the spleen due to splenic infarctions. (Image courtesy of Prof PJ Ell.)**

Fig. 1.21 **Anterior view of right chest and upper abdomen. Focal uptake is seen in an epigastric wound from recent peptic ulcer surgery.**

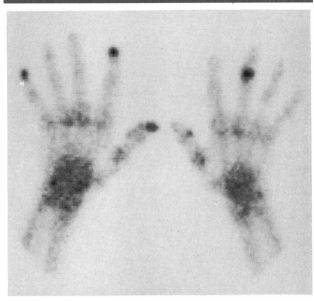

Fig. 1.22

Fig. 1.22 Calcinosis circumscripta of the hands producing focal hot spots in several digits. Accumulation of the bone scan agents suggests the process is still metabolically active.

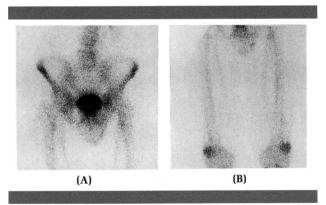

(A) (B)

Fig. 1.23 Increased tracer uptake in vessels on the anterior pelvic (A) and femoral (B) views due to vascular calcification.

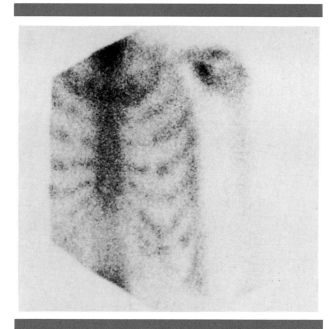

Fig. 1.24 **Tracer uptake in the costal cartilages due to calcification.**

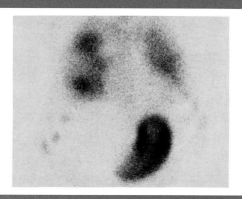

Fig. 1.25 **Anterior view of chest and upper abdomen in patient with prolonged hypercalcaemia. Diffuse tracer uptake is seen in the lung and stomach due to soft tissue calcification.**

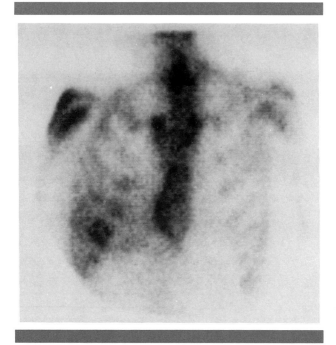

Fig. 1.26 **Anterior view of chest and upper abdomen in 58-year-old woman with severe longstanding rheumatoid arthritis. Diffuse liver uptake of tracer is seen due to amyloid infiltration. The right shoulder is hot due to arthritis.**

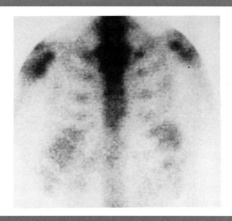

Fig. 1.27 Anterior view of chest and upper abdomen, showing increased uptake over both breasts in a 37-year-old woman. This is a normal variant.

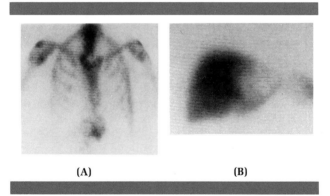

(A)   (B)

Fig. 1.28 (A) Anterior view of chest and upper abdomen from a patient with breast cancer showing tracer uptake in a hepatic metastasis. The colloid liver scan from the patient (B) confirms the presence of the liver metastasis.

Because of great sensitivity in detecting skeletal pathology, bone scanning has been extensively employed in the
study of patients with established or suspected bony malignant disease. The technique can be applied either to
bone metastases or to primary bony tumours.

BONE SCANS APPEARANCES
OF METASTASES

Malignant disease invading the skeleton normally excites
some osteoblastic response locally. This is true even in
most cases where the X-ray appearances are lytic. As a
result the characteristic bone scan appearance of a metastasis is as an area of increased tracer uptake, ie a 'hot spot'
(Fig. 2.1). Multiple metastases appear as irregularly distributed areas of increased tracer uptake (Fig. 2.2 A, B, C).
While sensitive for metastases the bone scan is non-specific. Thus, metastases from different sites have identical
appearances on the bone scan, so that the technique is of
no value in identifying an unknown primary malignancy
in a patient who presents with metastases.

Some tumours fail to excite an osteoblastic response
when they invade the skeleton. Fortunately this is rare and
the incidence of false negative bone scans in metastases
has been reported to be less than 3%. It is essential, however, to obtain skeletal X-rays of any site of bone pain
which is negative on bone scan to exclude the possibility
of such a false negative. The tumour most commonly associated with a false negative bone scan is myeloma. This
produces purely osteolytic lesions, a fact which correlates
with the finding that the serum alkaline phosphatase is
usually normal even when there is extensive skeletal involvement. In myeloma patients with extensive skeletal
disease the bone scan is seldom completely normal, but

the extent of disease revealed is often considerably less than on skeletal X-rays. Skeletal X-ray surveys rather than bone scans should thus be obtained in myelomatosis.

In patients with extensive metastases the individual lesions may coalesce to produce the so-called superscan appearance (Fig. 2.3 A–F). This consists of generally high tracer uptake in the skeleton, low soft tissue background activity and failure to visualize the kidneys. A similar appearance is seen in metabolic bone disease (see Chapter 4) but the metastatic superscan can usually be distinguished by the fact that tracer uptake in the skeleton is not usually completely uniform. Additionally, in a metastatic super-scan the skull and limbs do not usually show diffusely

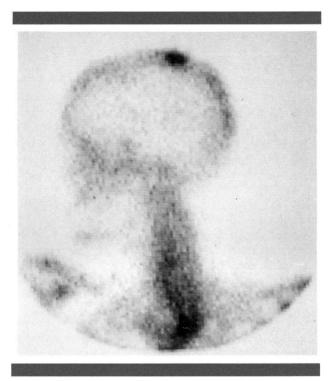

Fig. 2.1 **Left lateral skull view from 64-year-old woman with previous breast cancer. Focal 'hot spot' in vault of skull due to a metastasis.**

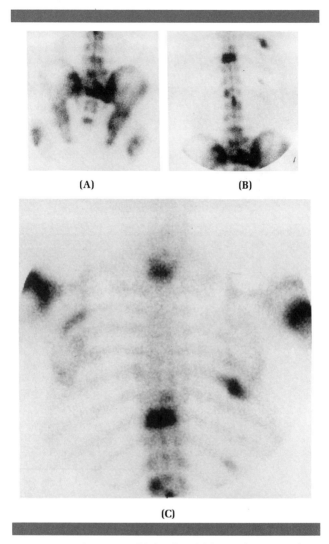

(A) (B)

(C)

Fig. 2.2 Posterior views of (A) pelvis (B) lower thoracic and lumbar spine and (C) thoracic spine and ribs from 68-year-old man with prostatic cancer. There are multiple hot spots in the upper femur, pelvis, sacrum, lumbar spine, thoracic spine, ribs and shoulders due to multiple focal metastases.

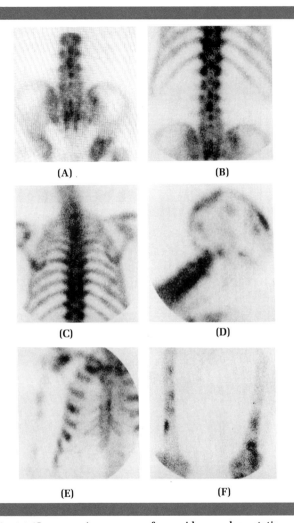

(A)

(B)

(C)

(D)

(E)

(F)

Fig. 2.3 'Superscan' appearance from widespread prostatic carcinoma metastases in a 72-year-old man. Diffusely increased uptake is seen in the pelvis, spine and posterior ribs (A, B and C) though some non-homogeneity of uptake is evident. Non-homogeneous uptake is more evident in the skull (D), anterior ribs (E) and femora (F), indicating the presence of metastases rather than metabolic bone disease as the cause of the superscan.

increased uptake, a finding which contrasts with metabolic bone disease. Any primary tumour can produce a metastatic superscan but it occurs most commonly in disseminated prostatic or breast cancer.

Metastatic lesions which fail to produce an osteoblastic reaction may, if large enough, be detected on the bone scan as 'cold spots' (Fig. 2.4). Up to 2% of metastases are cold on bone scanning. The primary tumours which have the highest frequency of cold metastases are renal carcinoma and melanoma but this appearance can be seen in any tumour. Hot and cold metastases may co-exist in the same

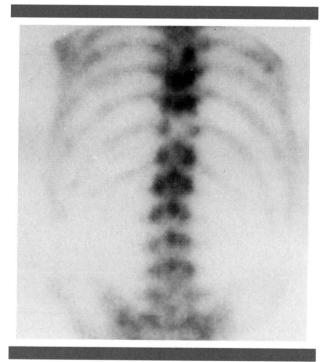

Fig. 2.4 **Posterior view of lumbar and lower thoracic spine from 63-year-old man with prostatic metastases. Increased uptake due to metastases is evident in lower thoracic and upper lumbar vertebrae, with the exception of T11 which shows decreased uptake due to metastastic involvement without osteoblastic reaction.**

patient and individual metastases may change their appearance during the course of the disease.

Because of the non-specificity of the bone scan the finding of an abnormal bone scan in a patient with malignant disease raises questions of whether the lesions are due to metastases or not. The intensity of uptake of tracer is no guide as to the likelihood of a lesion being malignant. Metastases, Paget's disease, trauma and infection may all cause markedly increased uptake on the bone scan while some tumours may cause only slightly increased uptake. The number of lesions can provide some guide as to likelihood of malignancy. Patients who have multiple focal lesions scattered throughout the skeleton are likely to have metastases, though the possibility of other causes should not be completely dismissed, especially if the patient's clinical state is against disseminated malignancy. Solitary bone lesions are especially difficult. Around 10–20% of patients who present with metastases will do so with a single bone scan abnormality. The site of the solitary abnormality has some bearing on the likelihood of malignancy. A single lesion in a periarticular region is likely to be benign, whereas a single lesion in the pedicle of a vertebra is highly likely to be malignant. In the case of single lesions a careful history of possible trauma should always be obtained, and X-rays of the area obtained followed by CT or MRI if necessary. Where doubt persists biopsy of the area may be indicated or a repeat bone scan obtained in several months' time. A recommended protocol for investigation of suspected metastases is shown in Fig. 2.5.

The distribution or shape of lesions may also help in deciding the likelihood of malignancy. A single focal abnormality in a rib (Fig. 2.6) is likely to be due to trauma, whereas a lesion extending along the rib (Fig. 2.7) is probably malignant. A series of focal rib lesions in a linear array (Fig. 2.8) is characteristic of trauma. Intense uniform involvement of a whole bone is characteristic of Paget's disease, but on occasions can be due to metastases, especially from prostatic cancer. Linear uptake in a vertebra, particularly when multiple vertebrae are involved, is usually due to benign collapse rather than malignancy (see Chapter 4).

It has recently been suggested that in patients with bone

Protocol for investigation of suspected skeletal metastases

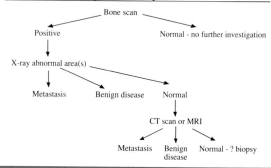

Fig. 2.5 **Suggested protocol for investigation of suspected metastases.**

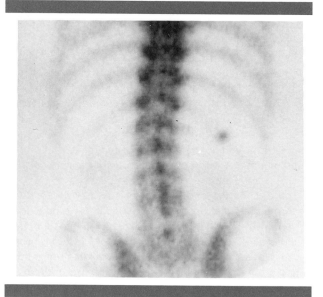

Fig. 2.6 **Single hot spot in right 12th rib of a 52-year-old woman with previous breast carcinoma. The bone scan was otherwise normal. A metastasis cannot be excluded from the scan, but, as in this patient, this appearance is often due to trauma.**

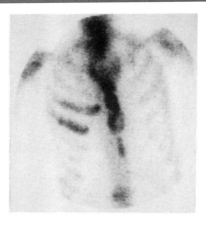

Fig. 2.7 **Anterior view of chest from 57-year-old man with disseminated lung cancer. The lesions extending along the right 3rd and 4th ribs are characteristic of metastatic involvement. Metastases are also evident in the sternum and thoracic spine.**

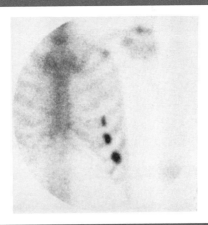

Fig. 2.8 **Anterior view of left chest from man with rib pain and previous carcinoma of prostate. Focally increased uptake in a linear array in three ribs is seen, characteristic of trauma.**

scan lesions of uncertain significance bone marrow scanning using ^{99m}Tc-nanocolloid may be helpful. This colloid is taken up intensely by the liver and spleen, obscuring uptake of tracer by the lower ribs and the lower thoracic and upper lumbar vertebrae. At other skeletal sites a bone scan lesion which is cold on nanocolloid imaging is likely to be malignant (Fig. 2.9 A, B), whereas bone scan lesions which show normal nanocolloid uptake are usually degenerative in nature.

Bone scanning for clinically suspected metastases

Bone metastases may be suspected because of bone pain, presence of metastases elsewhere in the body or because of biochemical abnormalities such as hypercalcaemia or an elevated serum alkaline phosphatase. In each of these situations the bone scan is an appropriate initial investigation to employ in detecting or confirming bone metastases.

The presence of bone pain in a patient with a current or previous extra-osseous malignancy is a sinister occurrence, but can be due to pathologies other than malignancy. A local X-ray of the area in question should be obtained but

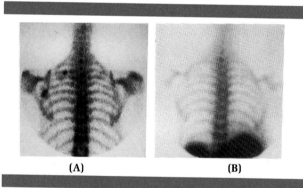

(A)   **(B)**

Fig. 2.9 **(A) Posterior rib and thoracic spine bone scan view from 69-year-old man with non-Hodgkin's lymphoma. Several hot spots are seen, due to bone involvement by tumour. (B) ^{99m}Tc nanocolloid bone marrow image from same patient. The bone scan hot spots in the left upper ribs are mirrored by decreased uptake on the marrow scan. (Images courtesy of Prof PJ Ell.)**

usually needs to be considered with a bone scan of the whole body. If the bone X-ray is negative the bone scan may reveal metastases because of its greater sensitivity. If the bone X-ray reveals metastatic disease at the symptomatic site, the bone scan is invaluable in demonstrating whether there are lesions elsewhere in the skeleton. This may be of crucial importance when planning ports for radiotherapy, as the result of the scan can indicate the need to extend the field to include lesions which are currently asymptomatic but potentially troublesome in the future. In patients with equivocal or subtle X-ray changes which may be due to metastases, the finding of a bone scan abnormality at the same site strengthens the case for considering a lesion to be significant.

In patients who have tumours with a high propensity to spread to bone, eg breast cancer or lung cancer, the presence of soft tissue metastases is an indication for obtaining a bone scan, as a significant proportion of patients will also have asymptomatic bone metastases. The presence of bony lesions will alter the prognosis and appropriate method of management in some cases.

Biochemical markers of bone metastases are often non-specific and provide no information on the site of the lesions. Hypercalcaemia in a cancer patient should lead to a bone scan, to detect the possible causative metastases. It should be noted, however, that there is often poor correlation between the degree of hypercalcaemia and the extent of metastases. In extreme cases hypercalcaemia may be present without any bone metastases being detected. This apparent discrepancy arises because of the ability of some tumours to produce polypeptide compounds which have parathyroid hormone-like qualities, resulting in metabolic rather than metastatic mobilization of calcium from the skeleton in addition to increased renal tubular reabsorption of calcium. An elevated serum alkaline phosphatase may be due to bone metastases, but other causes such as Paget's disease may be demonstrated on the bone scan.

Assessing the response of bone metastases to therapy
Successful radiotherapy for bone metastases will stop bony invasion by tumour. The local osteoblastic response will

die down and increased uptake will no longer be seen on the bone scan. Normal bone included in a radiotherapy field also has some impairment of osteoblastic activity and shows lower than normal uptake on a bone scan (Fig. 2.10). The bone scan appearances after X-ray therapy are characteristic.

Assessing the response of bone metastases to systemic therapy, such as cytotoxic drugs or hormonal manipulation, is more difficult. Patients who show fewer lesions on the post-therapy compared to pre-therapy bone scan are likely to have responded to the treatment (Fig. 2.11 A, B). By contrast, patients who show a more extensive lesion or an increased number of lesions on the post-therapy scan (Fig. 2.12 A, B) are likely to have progressive disease,

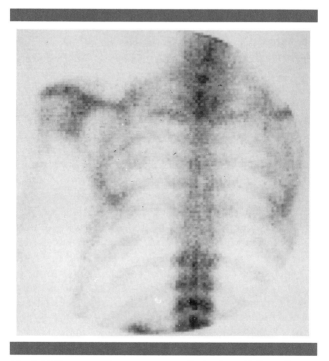

Fig. 2.10 **Decreased bone tracer uptake in the mid thoracic vertebrae and adjacent ribs due to X-ray therapy given nine months previously.**

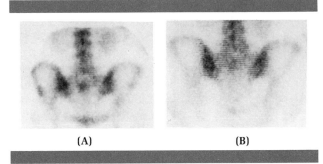

(A) (B)

Fig. 2.11 (A) Posterior view of pelvis and lower lumbar spine from 49-year-old woman with breast cancer. Hot spots in the sacrum, left sacro-iliac joint and pelvic bones due to metastases. (B) Repeat bone scan 12 months later after tamoxifen treatment. The sacral and left sacro-iliac lesions are just apparent but the remainder are no longer visible indicating regression of disease.

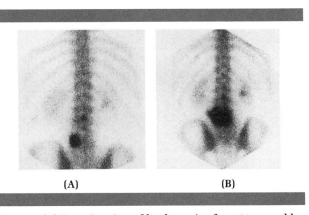

(A) (B)

Fig. 2.12 (A) Posterior view of lumbar spine from 61-year-old man with carcinoma of prostate showing metastases in L5. (B) Repeat study one year later shows a more extensive abnormality in L5 indicating progression of disease.

though care has to be taken to exclude the 'flare phenomenon'. The flare phenomenon occurs in the first few months after institution of systemic therapy for bone metastases. During this period metastases which are healing under the influence of the therapy may show a marked osteoblastic response. Apparently new lesions may even appear because of the healing of metastases which previously did not excite enough bone reaction to be visible on the scan. This change of appearance can easily be misinterpreted as a progression of disease. Because of the possibility of a flare phenomenon occurring, a follow-up bone scan assessing the response to therapy should be deferred for 6 months.

It is tempting to interpret changes in intensity of individual lesions in terms of disease progression. This is, however, unreliable. The intensity of uptake in lesions is dependent on many technical factors such as use of different cameras, photographic exposure etc. Furthermore, the time between injection of the radiopharmaceutical and imaging is crucial, with much evidence to show that the metastases-to-normal bone activity ratio increases with time from injection. The relationship between the metastases and the osteoblastic reaction in the surrounding bone is complex. Thus an increase in activity in a lesion on bone scan may indicate progression of disease exciting more osteoblastic response or may be due to healing of the lesion. Conversely, a decrease in activity may be due to slowing of growth of the metastases or to the onset of bony invasion that is so rapid that the osteoblastic response is unable to keep up. Because of the many, and often conflicting, factors which may produce a change of intensity of bone agent uptake, this parameter should not be used in deciding on response of bone metastases to therapy.

There has been considerable interest recently in the use of beta-radiation-emitting bone-seeking radionuclides for therapy of bone metastases. Strontium-89 (^{89}Sr) has undergone some initial studies. This radiopharmaceutical, like the diphosphonates, localizes in areas of osteoblastic activity and thus will produce increased uptake around most metastases and deliver local radiotherapy with relative sparing of normal bone and the bone marrow. Initial results with ^{89}Sr suggest a useful palliative effect on bone pain from metastases in most patients with prostatic cancer and perhaps also breast cancer. Some marrow toxicity is observed but is usually mild unless the patient has very extensive metastases and has had previous vigorous treatments with chemotherapy or radiotherapy. Further large trials with this agent are currently in progress. An alternative approach under investigation is the use of various diphosphonates labelled with beta-emitters such as yttrium-90, samarrium-153 or rhenium-168.

Bone scanning in the staging and follow-up of malignancy

While there is general agreement on the essential role of the bone scan in patients with symptoms of bone metastases, its place in the staging of cancer patients with no clinical evidence of bone metastases is much more controversial.

Bone scanning can be justified in asymptomatic patients if there is an adequate yield of positive studies, if the number of false positive studies is acceptably low and if the information generated either changes management or is prognostically significant. Considerable information is available on the use of bone scanning for routine staging in common tumours such as breast, lung or prostate cancer, and some consensus is now emerging. For most other tumours only a small number of series is available.

It has long been known that up to 85% of patients dying from breast cancer will show evidence of bone metastases. Because of this high figure and the frequency with which this tumour occurs, routine bone scanning has been studied most extensively in breast cancer. Several early studies reported a high incidence of bone scan abnormalities in patients with apparently early (clinical Stage I or II) breast cancer, with various series in the 1960s and early 1970s finding positivity rates of 15 to 40% in this group of patients. Such a high yield led to an initial enthusiasm for routine scanning in all patients presenting with breast cancer whatever the stage. It has subsequently become apparent that the true figures for bone metastases are much lower – probably less than 1% in Stage I and less than 3% in Stage II. The reasons for the higher incidence in the early studies is not entirely clear but may be due to inadequate selection of patients and a tendency to misinterpret bone scan abnormalities due to benign disease as metastases when the technique was new. The relatively low incidence of bone metastases in asymptomatic patients with early breast cancer has made the case for routine scanning less clear-cut.

Currently there is no overall agreement on whether all patients with early breast cancer should have bone scans. In some centres every patient with early breast cancer has a bone scan carried out on the basis that this gives prognostic information and serves as a baseline for comparison if future bone scans are required. Other centres are more selective and reserve bone scanning for those early breast cancer patients who exhibit adverse prognostic features such as tumour involvement on axillary node sampling or an unfavourable oestrogen receptor status. The authors' view is that routine bone scanning is not justified in Stage I but is useful in Stage II. Patients with clinically more advanced disease (Stages III and IV) demonstrate a high incidence of bone metastases even when asymptomatic and routine scanning at presentation is justifiable. All patients being entered into clinical trials of therapies for breast cancer should have a bone scan, whatever their clinical stage.

The role of the bone scan in the follow-up patients treated for breast cancer is also a matter of debate. The bone scan may show certain changes as a result of breast surgery. Trauma to the underlying ribs during mastectomy may lead to focal hot spots which can persist for several months while loss of attenuation by removal of the breast may make the ribs on that side appear more prominent. Avascular necrosis or rib fractures after radiotherapy may also cause bone scan changes. It is essential to bear these possibilities in mind when interpreting bone scans in post-mastectomy patients. In most centres bone scans are now obtained in post-mastectomy patients only if they have clinical or biochemical evidence of bone metastases or if there is a local or other soft tissue recurrence of disease. In some centres, on the other hand, routine bone scans are obtained at regular (eg annual) intervals whether the patient has symptoms or not.

Bone metastases are found at autopsy in up to 50% of patients with lung cancer. Bone scans at presentation are abnormal in around 30% of patients with lung cancer, and are associated with an adverse prognosis. If only patients with potentially operable lung cancer are considered, the rate of positive bone scans at presentation falls to between 4% and 20% in various series. Because of the high morbidity and mortality associated with lung cancer surgery it is worthwhile identifying patients who have bone metastases as attempts at operative cure in this group are futile. For this reason, even at a pick-up rate of only 4% a routine bone scan can be justified pre-operatively in all patients. It is essential, however, that each patient with a positive bone scan should be further investigated by radiology or bone biopsy to confirm the presence of bone metastases before excluding them from surgical resection, as this is currently the only treatment with any chance of a cure.

Bone scans at presentation in lung cancer can also be useful in identifying the presence of local bone invasion by the tumour, and can be especially helpful in Pancoast tumours (Fig. 2.13 A, B) by showing changes before the bone radiographs become abnormal. The bone scan abnormalities can, on occasions, be subtle and once again confirmation of the nature of the bone scan lesion should be

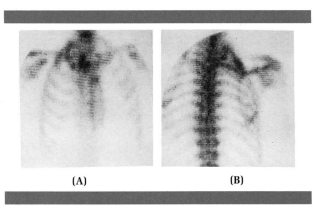

(A)   (B)

Fig. 2.13 **Bone scan from 59-year-old man with right apical bronchial carcinoma demonstrating local involvement of the upper ribs both anteriorly (A) and posteriorly (B). The posterior view also shows an area of decreased uptake in the second rib due to bone destruction.**

obtained before making management decisions about the patient.

Routine bone scanning during follow-up is not justified in lung cancer because of the relatively short average survival and the lack of an effective, non-toxic therapy for asymptomatic bone metastases. They should, of course, be obtained when clinically indicated by symptoms.

Characteristic bone scan changes are also seen in hypertrophic pulmonary osteoarthropathy (HPOA, Fig. 2.14). The bone scan changes of HPOA frequently appear before X-rays become abnormal.

In prostatic cancer up to 70% of patients have evidence of bone metastases at autopsy. Studies on bone scanning at presentation have suggested that 30–50% of unselected patients have bone metastases at this time. When classified by stage the rate of positivity appears to be around 5% for Stage I, 10% for Stage II and 20% for Stage III. Several series have demonstrated that the bone scan is more sensitive than serum acid or alkaline phosphatase levels for detecting bone metastases. It has also been shown that patients with a positive bone scan at presentation have a considerably higher mortality at two years than those with normal scans. In view of the relatively high yield, the useful prognostic information and the possibility of hormonal manipulation of the tumour, bone scans should be

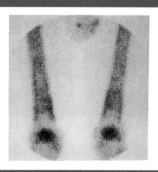

Fig. 2.14 **Bone scan of femora from 66-year-old man with lung cancer. There is increased cortical uptake characteristic of hypertrophic pulmonary osteoarthropathy.**

obtained in all patients presenting with prostatic cancer. The use of routine bone scanning in the follow-up of patients with prostatic cancer is less clear-cut. A number of patients will convert from negative to positive during follow-up but it is uncertain how much additional information can be obtained by routine scanning as opposed to using biochemical markers for bone metastases.

Melanoma shows a propensity to spread to bone, but at presentation the frequency of bone metastases is low in Stage I or II patients, and bone scans should be reserved for patients with clinically more advanced disease or some clinical indication of metastases. Melanoma can produce lytic metastases on occasions and bone X-rays should always be obtained of painful sites, even when the bone scan is negative.

In gynaecological cancer only a small number of series have been published. Patients with clinically early cervical (Stage 0, I or II) or ovarian (Stage I or II) cancer showed a low incidence of positive bone scans and routine bone scanning at presentation is not justified. The position is more questionable in patients with clinically advanced disease. In endometrial cancer the frequency of positive bone scans at presentation is low and only patients with symptoms of bone metastases should be studied.

Though renal carcinoma has a recognized tendency to spread to bone, the frequency of abnormal bone scans at presentation is low, and bone scanning cannot be justified in the absence of symptoms suggesting metastases. The same policy should be adopted in bladder cancer, thyroid cancer, gastrointestinal tract tumours and haematological malignancies.

BONE SCANNING IN PRIMARY BONE TUMOURS

The isotope bone scan is not a reliable technique for the differential diagnosis of primary bone tumours – this usually depends on a combination of bone radiology and biopsy. The bone scan can, however, be a useful adjunctive technique. Intensity of uptake does not differentiate between benign and malignant primary bone tumours, though a lesion which does not show increased tracer uptake is unlikely to be malignant. Similarly, a lesion which shows marked vascularity on a three phase bone scan is likely to be malignant (Fig. 2.15 A, B). In the case of radiologically dubious tumours a bone scan can be valuable in demonstrating that the abnormality is metabolically active, though increased uptakes does not prove it is malignant.

Some reports have appeared of scintigraphic appearances which are typical of individual primary bone tumours. The overlap in bone scan findings in different bone malignancies is, however, too great for this to be of any real clinical value.

In osteogenic sarcoma, the role of the bone scan in determining the extent of the primary tumour is controversial. While some studies have found good correlation between the bone scan abnormality and the resected specimen, others have suggested that the scan may overestimate the proximal extent of the tumour, probably because of increased vascularity. The bone scan is also unable to demonstrate intramedullary or any soft tissue extension of the primary lesion. For these reasons CT or MRI is more accurate in the pre-operative assessment of the primary tumour.

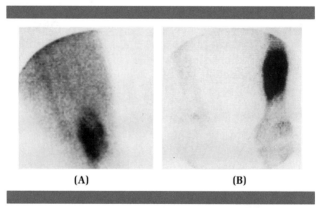

(A) **(B)**

Fig. 2.15 **(A) Blood pool and (B) delayed bone scan images from a 27-year-old man with a poorly differentiated sarcoma of the lower left femur. The lesion is highly vascular and shows intense uptake on the delayed images.**

The main role of the bone scan in osteogenic sarcoma is in the detection of distant bone metastases. At the time of presentation the incidence of distant bone metastases is low at around 2%. In view of the aggressive nature of surgical treatment of primary osteosarcoma (amputation or resection and limb reconstruction) it is worthwhile detecting the small number of patients who present with bony metastases as this finding may modify treatment. It is, of course, essential to confirm that bone scan abnormalities are indeed due to metastases.

In follow-up of patients treated with adjuvant chemotherapy bone scanning is of value in showing bone metastases, which may be the first indication of recurrence and some centres employ routine bone scanning during follow-up for this reason.

Soft tissue metastases from osteosarcoma may demonstrate uptake of bone scan agents (Fig. 2.16). Such uptake should always be sought in osteosarcoma patients having a bone scan; but the technique cannot be used as a primary screening method for soft tissue recurrence, as failure of bone scan agent uptake is frequent enough to make the technique unreliable.

In Ewing's sarcoma the frequency of distant bone metastases is around 10% and the bone scan should be used in the initial staging of all patients with this tumour. Bone metastases also frequently develop during follow-up and may be the first site of recurrence. This has led to some centres performing regular bone scans during follow-up. Soft tissue metastases from Ewing's sarcoma do not take up bone scan agents, and cannot be detected on the bone scan. Gallium-67 citrate does, however, show uptake in these lesions and may be valuable in demonstrating them.

Osteosarcoma may also develop in association with Paget's disease, though only rarely. Paget's disease itself causes increased uptake and the sarcoma usually has less avidity for the bone scan agent. The scan appearance is thus one of relatively decreased uptake within the hot lesion of pagetic bone. If ^{67}Ga is given, by contrast, the sarcoma will show higher uptake than the Paget's disease. Osteosarcoma complicating Paget's disease should be suspected if the bone scan shows increased uptake projecting

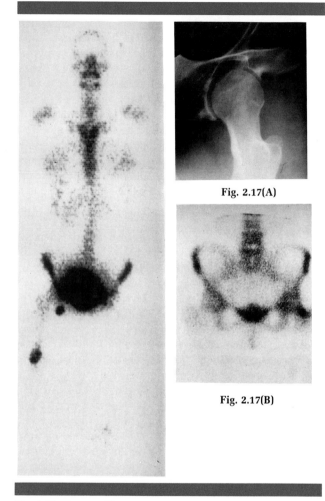

Fig. 2.17(A)

Fig. 2.17(B)

Fig. 2.16 **22-year-old woman with right above-knee amputation for osteosarcoma of lower femur two years previously. There is increased uptake in the right groin due to a lymph node metastasis and in the tip of the femoral stump due to local recurrence.**

Fig. 2.17 **(A) X-ray of left hip and (B) anterior bone scan of pelvis and upper femora in 25-year-old man with osteoid osteoma of left femoral neck. The X-ray was interpreted as normal. The bone scan shows a focus of intense uptake in the left femoral neck.**

out with the main mass of the bone or crossing a joint space in an irregular fashion.

The frequency of distant bone metastases at presentation in chondrosarcoma is not established. The bone scan may prove useful in demonstrating lesions not seen on skeletal X-rays. This appears to be especially the case in spinal lesions which account for around 6% of primary chrondrosarcomas.

The benign bone tumour in which bone scanning has the best recognized role is osteoid osteoma. This tumour usually produces a small oval or round area of lucency surrounded by sclerosis on X-ray, but such changes are not always detectable, especially in the spine. The characteris-

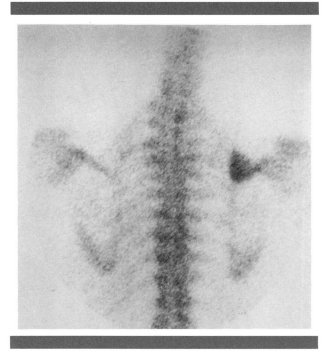

Fig. 2.18 **Posterior view of thoracic spine and ribs from a 50-year-old man with an enchondroma of the right scapula. An area of markedly increased uptake is seen at the site of the lesion. (Image courtesy of Prof PJ Ell.)**

tic bone scan appearance is a highly localized area of markedly increased tracer uptake (Fig. 2.17 A, B). A central, colder area is sometimes seen with the lesion. The bone scan is much more sensitive than X-ray for osteoid osteoma and a normal bone scan essentially excludes this diagnosis. In a patient with a history suggestive of osteoid osteoma a bone X-ray of the affected area should be obtained followed by a bone scan if this is negative. In some centres the bone scan has also been used to locate the lesion at surgery. Two hours prior to surgery the patient is given a small dose of ^{99m}Tc-MDP and a sterilized probe is then used to detect the site of high activity in the bone. This technique may be of value in demonstrating that the tumour has been completely excised by the surgeon.

It should be noted that increased uptake may be seen with other benign bone tumours (Fig. 2.18).

The bone scan has an important role in the study of patients with suspected osteomyelitis, especially in the early phase of the disease. The combination of bone scanning with either Gallium-67 citrate or labelled white cell imaging can increase sensitivity and specificity, especially in more chronic forms of infection.

PATHOLOGY OF ACUTE OSTEOMYELITIS

Bone infection may arise either by direct spread from adjacent soft tissue or joint infection or by blood-borne spread from a distant site of infection. Haematogenous osteomyelitis can occur at any age and be due to a wide variety of organisms, but is most often seen in children and is most commonly due to *Staphylococcus aureus*. In children the condition is most often present in the metaphyses of long bones where the nutrient artery gives rise to multiple channels which flow towards the epiphysis (growth plate). On the metaphyseal side of the growth plate the channels turn back on themselves to empty into large sinusoidal veins. The slow flow within these vessels produces an ideal site for multiplication of bacteria. In the child the looping back of vessels in this fashion protects the epiphyses and the ends of the long bones. In the adult, and in the infant, the nutrient arteries do not loop back and infection is not so confined to the metaphyseal area.

The initial process in acute osteomyelitis appears to be local oedema which causes elevation of the periosteum and impaired blood flow with resultant necrosis of bone. The characteristic radiographic changes of periosteal elevation and bone destruction are rarely seen earlier than 10–12 days after the onset of symptoms.

Bone scan appearances in acute osteomyelitis

As discussed in Chapter 1, three phase bone scanning is often employed in suspected osteomyelitis. The ^{99m}Tc-diphosphonate is injected as a bolus with the symptomatic area under the gamma camera. A dynamic flow study is obtained, at usually 2 seconds per frame for up to 60 seconds. Whenever possible normal bone (eg the contralateral limb) should also be imaged for comparison. A blood pool image is obtained at 5–10 minutes post-injection. Standard static images are then performed at 3–4 hours. As a rule static images should be obtained of the whole skeleton in acute osteomyelitis, as other sites of infection in the skeleton may be discovered.

The typical bone scan findings in acute osteomyelitis are of increased blood flow and blood pool and markedly increased uptake on the static images (Fig. 3.1 A, B, C). The three phase bone scan helps to distinguish osteomyelitis from soft tissue infection adjacent to the bone. Soft tissue infection will give rise to increased flow and blood pool due to hyperaemia. In the absence of bone infection and resultant osteoblastic reaction, the increased uptake on the static images in soft tissue infection is, however, only slight (Fig. 3.2 A, B, C).

In the very early stages of acute osteomyelitis, the occlusion of the nutrient vessels by thrombosis and pressure of local oedema will cause a decrease in blood flow and an area of reduced activity may be seen on both the flow and static images (see Fig. 7.11, page 130). However, in practice, this appearance is seldom seen and, as described above, one normally finds increased uptake. The bone scan changes in osteomyelitis may be subtle, especially in the early stages. Furthermore, in children, abnormalities are frequently found close to the increased uptake of the epiphyseal plate and additional views are often required, particularly the use of magnification by converging or pinhole collimators. The bone scan is characteristically abnormal within 48 hours of the onset of symptoms in contrast with the 10–12 days after symptoms when radiographic changes become apparent.

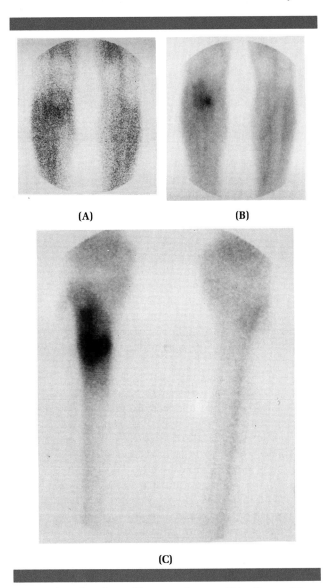

(A)

(B)

(C)

Fig. 3.1 **Anterior views of knees and upper tibiae from a 29-year-old man with osteomyelitis of the right upper tibia. Characteristically increased uptake is seen on the dynamic or flow (A), blood pool (B) and static images (C).**

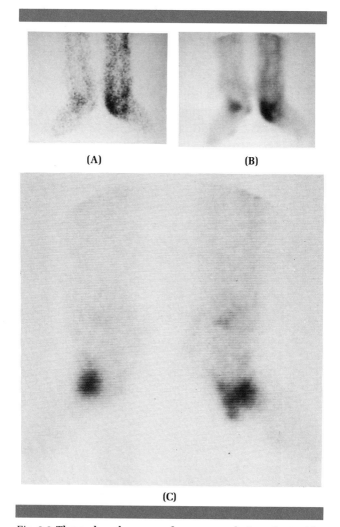

(A)

(B)

(C)

Fig. 3.2 **Three-phase bone scan from a paraplegic patient with extensive soft tissue infection of the lower legs and osteomyelitis of the right talus and left calcaneum. The areas of osteomyelitis show intensely increased uptake on the flow (A), blood pool (B) and static images (C). The soft tissue infection shows markedly increased uptake on the flow and blood pool images but only slightly increased uptake on the static image.**

ROLE OF THE BONE SCAN IN ACUTE OSTEOMYELITIS

Many studies have now been published documenting the very high sensitivity of the bone scan in acute osteomyelitis – most showing sensitivity figures in excess of 90%. Some difficulties may be encountered in neonates (see Chapter 7) and patients on steroids may show an increased frequency of false negative studies. In the paediatric age group specificity has also proved to be high, though some false positive results due to other pathologies, such as tumour, are seen. The problem of specificity increases with age and in adults the proportion of false positive studies is higher. As noted above, three phase bone scanning can improve specificity somewhat by helping to differentiate soft tissue infection from osteomyelitis.

The use of Gallium-67 citrate or labelled leucocyte imaging can also be of value. ^{67}Ga citrate has an affinity both for tumour and for inflammatory processes by mechanisms which are not yet fully understood. The tracer is given by i.v. injection and images are obtained from 24 to 72 hours later. In osteomyelitis ^{67}Ga images may demonstrate soft tissue infection not apparent from the bone scan (Fig. 3.3 A, B).

Labelled leucocyte imaging can be performed using either an ^{111}In or ^{99m}Tc radiopharmaceutical. The leucocytes are separated in vitro from 25–50 ml of the patient's own blood by gravity centrifugation. In the case of ^{111}In oxine, which remains the most commonly employed radiopharmaceutical, the cells have to be suspended in saline rather than plasma because of the great affinity of the tracer for the plasma protein transferrin. When using ^{99m}Tc HMPAO the cells can be maintained in plasma. Both radiopharmaceuticals are non-selective cell labels by virtue of their lipid solubility so it is essential to remove red blood cells prior to labelling. A short period of incubation with the tracer is adequate to obtain satisfactory cell labelling. After washing to remove unbound radiopharmaceutical, the labelled cells are re-injected into the patient. With ^{99m}Tc-labelled cells imaging can be carried out at 4 hours. With ^{111}In-labelled cells positive results can be obtained at 4 hours but it is often necessary to obtain further images at

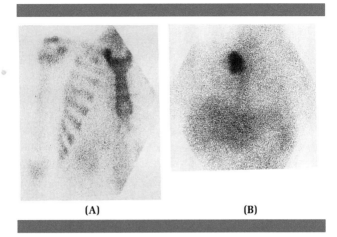

(A)   (B)

Fig. 3.3 **(A) Bone scan image of right anterior chest in 26-year-old man with osteomyelitis of the right second rib, which shows a small area of increased uptake anteriorly. (B) ^{67}Ga image of anterior chest in the same patient shows intensely increased uptake due to osteomyelitis and associated soft tissue infection. (Images provided by Dr SEM Clarke.)**

24 hours to show infection and a negative ^{111}In study at 4 hours does not exclude infection.

The characteristic appearance of acute osteomyelitis with labelled white cells is a focal area of increased tracer uptake which is clearly identifiable against the normal uptake of labelled cells in the marrow (Fig. 3.4 A, B, C, D). Some recent reports have suggested that care has to be exercised when interpreting ^{99m}Tc-labelled white cell studies as normal variation in the distribution of the marrow may produce apparent hot spots. The use of ^{99m}Tc nanocolloid marrow scanning may help to resolve this problem. Similar difficulties have not been encountered with ^{111}In-labelled cells, possibly because of the much lower injected activity and resultant poor count statistics and also the poorer resolution obtained because of the higher energy of ^{111}In.

In a patient who presents with suspected acute osteomyelitis a bone X-ray of the affected part should be obtained first. If this is normal, or equivocal, a three phase

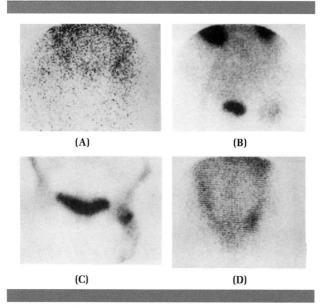

(A)

(B)

(C)

(D)

Fig. 3.4 **Three phase bone scan from a 63-year-old woman with postoperative osteomyelitis of the left femoral neck shows increased uptake on the flow (A), blood pool (B) and delayed images (C). These appearances could also be due to trauma. Focally increased uptake on the ^{111}In leucocyte image (D) makes infection very likely.**

bone scan should be obtained next. If the bone scan is negative, further investigation will depend on the clinical context. If the suspicion of osteomyelitis is not high, then observation and perhaps a repeat X-ray, then bone scan in 4 or 5 days would be appropriate. If, however, there is still a strong suspicion of osteomyelitis the choice lies between ^{67}Ga imaging, labelled leucocyte imaging, magnetic resonance imaging (where available) and fine needle aspiration. There is some doubt about the efficacy of the bone scan in detecting acute osteomyelitis in neonates, with some early studies demonstrating a lower sensitivity than that found in older children. With careful studies employing magnification procedures on modern, high resolution imaging equipment, the sensitivity in neonates may rise somewhat. This, however, remains a more difficult group in whom meticulous attention to detail and careful scrutiny for minor changes are particularly important.

The diabetic foot is another situation which may prove problematical. In this group of patients arthropathy and soft tissue infection are common. In the extreme case of a Charcot's joint markedly increased tracer uptake may be seen on the bone scan. Three phase bone scanning is only partially successful in distinguishing osteomyelitis from other pathologies in these patients. In the authors' experience labelled leucocyte imaging is the most reliable technique.

It is essential to realize that the bone scan is of no value in deciding when antibiotic therapy can be stopped in a patient with acute osteomyelitis, as bone repair will produce an abnormal study long after infection has settled. Persistence or absence of abnormal uptake of ^{67}Ga or labelled leucocytes may be of considerable value in this situation.

In patients who present with septicaemia (especially staphylococcal) from an unknown primary site of infection a bone scan is of value in looking for occult osteomyelitis.

Chronic osteomyelitis

Bone scan abnormalities may persist for a prolonged period after an episode of acute osteomyelitis, due to repair processes within the bone. Bone repair predominantly causes increased tracer uptake on the static images, but associated hyperaemia may also produce some flow and blood pool image abnormalities. For these reasons the bone scan alone is a poor guide to continuing presence of infection, though a normal bone scan usually means that the infection has settled.

Gallium-67 imaging is abnormal in chronic osteomyelitis. The intensity of uptake may be of some value in identifying patients with persistence or recurrence of acute infection though this is not universally accepted. A number of series have suggested that labelled leucocyte imaging is more reliable, and that continued labelled white cell accumulation at the site of osteomyelitis is a good pointer to continuing infection.

In patients with low grade bone infection (eg tuberculosis) an abnormal bone scan is found (Fig. 3.5). Such lesions usually also show ⁶⁷Ga uptake (Fig. 3.6 A, B).

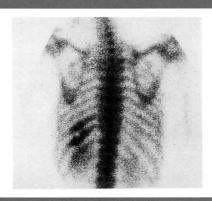

Fig. 3.5 **Bone scan of thoracic spine and posterior ribs from 33-year-old Asian man with tuberculous osteomyelitis of the ribs. Increased tracer uptake is seen along the posterior aspects of the left 10th and 11th ribs, the site of the disease.**

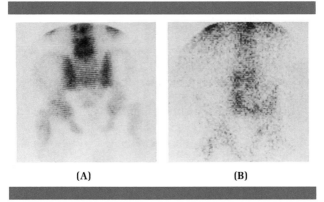

(A)   **(B)**

Fig. 3.6 **(A) Bone scan of lower lumbar spine and posterior pelvis from a 46-year-old diabetic, showing increased vertebral uptake due to tuberculous osteomyelitis. (B) Anterior ⁶⁷Ga image from the same patient shows increased bony uptake at the same site, plus adjacent soft tissue uptake due to a cold abscess.**

Periprosthetic infection

Prosthetic joints, and other orthopaedic appliances, provide a ready site for infection. The infection is often low grade, may present many months or years after insertion of the device and give rise to symptoms which are difficult to differentiate from those produced by mechanical problems such as loosening. When periprosthetic infection occurs, there is usually also some loosening present. This makes radiographic detection difficult.

Both infection and loosening will produce local accumulation of ^{99m}Tc-diphosphonate which is absent in a normal prosthesis. There is some debate, however, as to whether the pattern of uptake can allow the two processes to be separated. If a three phase study is performed an infected prosthesis will usually be associated with increased flow and blood pool (Fig. 3.7 A, B, C). A similar picture, however, may be seen in up to one third of patients with loosening and no evidence of infection. On the static images some authors have reported that diffuse increased uptake around the prosthesis (Fig. 3.8) was suggestive of infection while more focal uptake indicated loosening (Figs. 3.9 and 3.10). Other series, however, have indicated that the diffuse pattern is completely non-specific and concluded the bone scan alone is of no value in distinguishing between the two processes. The bone scan may also be of value in identifying the presence of heterotopic calcification (Fig. 3.11 A, B) or of an unsuspected fracture. It should be noted, however, that in the first year after joint replacement abnormalities may be related to surgery itself.

The use of combined bone and ^{67}Ga scanning has also been described in patients with suspected periprosthetic infection. ^{67}Ga imaging alone is of limited value, as loosening by itself can cause increased uptake of the tracer. Intense focal uptake of ^{67}Ga, however, favours infection (Fig. 3.12 A, B). In some series the presence of infection has been indicated by abnormality of the ^{67}Ga uptake which did not match the abnormal uptake of the bone scan agent – the so-called non-congruent pattern (Fig. 3.13 A, B) – whereas congruent uptake of the two radiopharmaceuticals was associated with loosening. Other series, however,

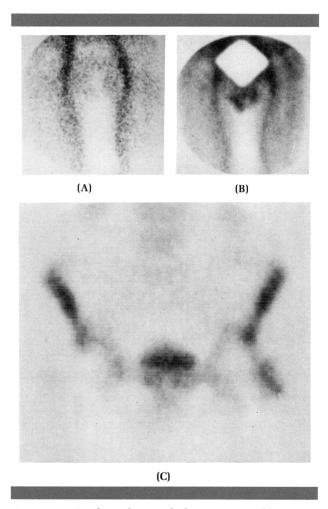

(A)   (B)

(C)

Fig. 3.7 Anterior three phase study from a 65-year-old patient with an infected left hip prosthesis. Increased uptake is noticed on the flow (A), blood pool (B) and static images (C). The right hip prosthesis is normal.

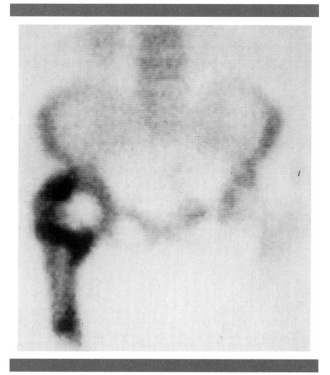

Fig. 3.8 **Anterior pelvic view from a 78-year-old woman with an infected right hip prosthesis. There is diffusely increased uptake around the prosthesis, suggesting infection.**

have found that some cases with congruent uptake had periprosthetic infection.

Labelled leucocyte imaging has also been employed. Abnormal white cell uptake around the prosthesis is specific for infection. The changes are often subtle, presumably due to the low grade inflammation present. False negative studies also occur and a negative labelled leucocyte study does not exclude the presence of infection.

In summary, therefore, the value of radionuclide techniques in differentiating between infection and loosening remains somewhat controversial. It is true, however, that a normal bone scan makes infection unlikely while diffuse uptake on the bone scan and either intense focal or incon-

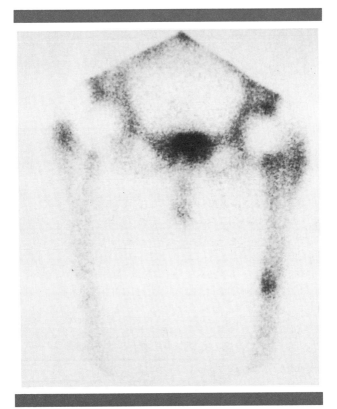

Fig. 3.9 **Anterior view of pelvis from a 63-year-old woman with bilateral hip prostheses and pain in the left hip. Increased uptake focally at the tip of the left prosthesis and in the intertrochanteric area, due to loosening of the prosthesis.**

gruent gallium uptake are very suggestive of periprosthetic infection. Accumulation of labelled leucocytes around the prosthesis appears to be fairly specific for infection but sensitivity remains debatable.

Septic arthritis
Patients with septic arthritis may develop osteomyelitis in the periarticular region due to direct spread from the infected joint. The clinical detection of bone involvement is difficult and bone scanning has been employed. The pres-

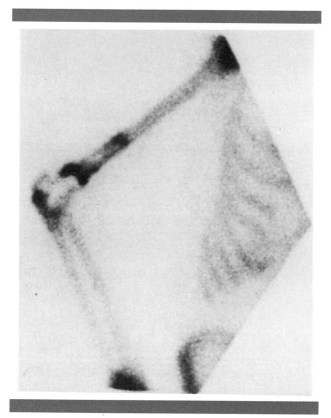

Fig. 3.10 **Bone scan of the right elbow from a 62-year-old woman with rheumatoid arthritis and a loose elbow prosthesis. There is increased uptake around the prosthesis, more marked at the tip of the prosthesis and the middle of the shaft. There is also increased uptake at the tip of the olecranon process.**

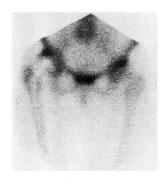

(A)

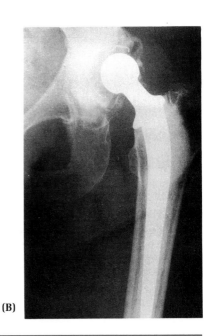

(B)

Fig. 3.11 **(A) Bone scan of upper femora from a 59-year-old woman with a left hip prosthesis. There is a single focal abnormality in the upper portion of the left acetabulum. This correlates with a site of new bone formation on X-ray (B), representing heterotopic calcification.**

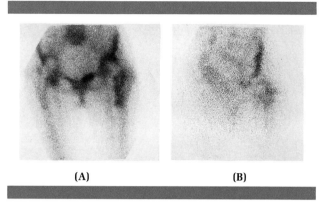

Fig. 3.12 **(A) Anterior bone scan of upper femora from a 78-year-old man with bilateral hip replacements and pyrexia of known origin. There is focally increased uptake around the femoral component of the right prosthesis and more diffusely increased uptake around the acetabular and femoral components of the left prosthesis. The ⁶⁷Ga image (B) shows localized uptake around the left upper femur, which was the site of periprosthetic infection.**

ence of joint infection by itself can produce bone scan abnormalities, with diffusely increased uptake in the periarticular bone on both sides of the affected joint. This appearance is thought to be due to hyperaemia induced by the joint infection. However, there have been reports of some patients with osteomyelitis secondary to joint infection having diffusely increased uptake of this type, so that such appearances do not exclude bone infection. More focally increased uptake is highly suggestive of osteomyelitis. Focally increased uptake of ⁶⁷Ga or labelled white cells within bone clearly favour osteomyelitis.

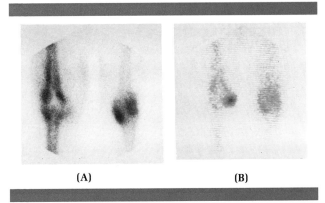

(A) (B)

Fig. 3.13 (A) Anterior bone scan of knees from a 51-year-old woman with rheumatoid arthritis and a right knee replacement. There is increased uptake in the left knee due to arthritis and diffusely increased uptake around the right knee prosthesis. (B) ^{67}Ga scan shows increased uptake in the left knee due to the inflammatory arthropathy. There is also focally increased uptake on the medial aspect of the right knee. This is discordant from the bone scan appearances and reflects periprosthetic infection at this site. (Images courtesy of Dr SEM Clarke.)

4 Bone Scanning and Photon Absorptiometry in Metabolic Bone Disease

While the exact mechanism by which ^{99m}Tc-diphosphonates localize in the skeleton is not fully understood, as discussed in Chapter 1, it is believed that they adsorb onto bone surfaces, most probably via the calcium in hydroxyapatite crystals. There is a particular predilection for sites of active bone formation and the major factors which affect adsorption are osteoblastic activity, and to a lesser extent, skeletal vascularity. It is therefore apparent that a bone scan image provides a functional display of skeletal metabolic activity.

Many of the metabolic bone diseases, with the exception of osteoporosis, are characterized by high bone turnover and are often associated with elevated levels of parathyroid hormone which causes increased bone resorption. As there is direct coupling between bone resorption and formation, an osteoblastic response follows osteoclastic activity, leading to new bone formation and increased affinity for ^{99m}Tc-diphosphonate. However, osteomalacia presents something of a paradox. This condition results from vitamin D deficiency, which produces a profound mineralization defect. In severe cases there is a massive excess of osteoid present with markedly reduced mineralization. Yet in this situation there is extremely high affinity for bone-seeking tracers. A possible explanation is that although there is excess osteoid with reduced mineralization, there is so much osteoid which is mineralizing, albeit slowly, that the total area of mineralization in the skeleton is in fact increased, even though the rate at any individual site is reduced.

Nevertheless, the bulk of evidence to date does suggest that bone uptake of tracer reflects skeletal metabolism and that this is likely to be primarily due to parathyroid hormone effects. Certainly, from clinical experience one has a strong impression that the bone scan appearances in metabolic bone disease reflect the degree of hyperparathyroidism that is present. The bone scan appearances in metabolic disease, however, are often non-specific and detection of abnormality depends upon a subjective impression of increased tracer uptake throughout the whole skeleton. Slightly increased tracer uptake throughout the skeleton may be virtually impossible to detect on the bone scan by visual inspection alone, and while quantitative techniques can be of value, these are not frequently performed. However, in the more severe cases of metabolic bone disease, the bone scan appearances can be quite dramatic and essentially diagnostic.

APPEARANCES IN METABOLIC BONE DISEASE

While the bone scan appearances in metabolic bone disease are non-specific, it is recognized that certain patterns of bone scan abnormality are commonly seen. The following metabolic features are characteristically seen in situations where increased skeletal metabolism exists:

1. Increased tracer uptake in the axial skeleton (Fig. 4.1)
2. Increased tracer uptake in the long bones
3. Increased tracer uptake in periarticular areas
4. Faint or absent kidney images (Fig. 4.1)
5. Prominent calvaria and mandible (Fig. 4.2)
6. 'Beading' of the costochondral junctions (Fig. 4.3)
7. 'Tie' sternum (Fig. 4.3)

The 'typical' bone scan finding in metabolic bone disease is a study that appears to be of excellent quality, with extremely good skeletal visualization. There is high contrast between bone and adjacent soft tissues. Any or all of the metabolic features listed above may be seen, reflecting increased bone uptake of tracer. Usually, the assessment of increased tracer uptake is a matter of subjective judgement. Nevertheless, in the calvaria and mandible, appearances may, on occasion be particularly prominent and produce striking images which are clearly recognizable as abnormal.

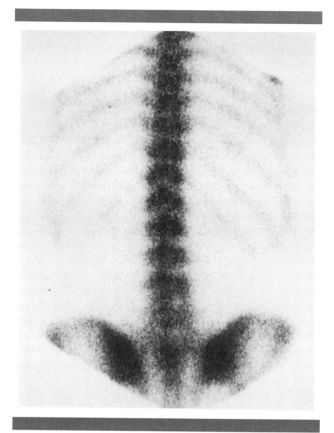

Fig. 4.1 **Posterior view of thoracolumbar spine showing diffusely increased uptake of tracer throughout. Note the renal images are not visualized.**

Indeed, in the most severe cases, appearances may be virtually pathognomonic of hyperparathyroidism (Fig. 4.2); whether primary or due to secondary causes such as renal disease òr osteomalacia. When there is generally increased skeletal avidity for tracer, the kidney images may appear faint, or even absent, due to the heightened contrast between bone and the kidneys, and with less tracer being available for excretion. Focally increased tracer uptake may be seen at the costochondral junctions, and the appearance has

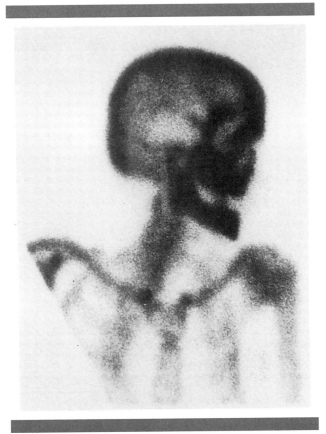

Fig. 4.2 **Lateral view of skull showing striking increased uptake of tracer throughout calvarium and mandible. Such dramatic appearances are found only with severe hyperparathyroidism. Note the increased uptake of tracer in clavicles and upper humeri.**

been referred to as 'beading' or the 'rosary bead' appearance. In the sternum there may be a general increase of tracer uptake by the manubrium and, in particular, the lateral borders of the body (the 'tie' sternum).

Renal osteodystrophy

In patients with severe renal osteodystrophy one may see

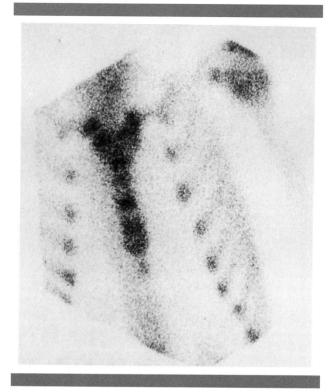

Fig. 4.3 **View of left anterior chest showing costochondral 'beading' and a 'tie' sternum.**

the most striking bone scan appearances found in the various metabolic bone disorders. There is markedly increased tracer uptake throughout the axial and peripheral skeleton and, in keeping with this, the kidneys appear faint and are frequently not visualized. There is extremely high contrast between bone and soft tissues, and the overall effect is to produce a so-called superscan image. The skull appearances may be virtually pathognomonic of severe hyperparathyroidism. Beading of the costochondral junctions and a tie sternum are also commonly seen. It is probable that most of the scan findings are due to increased bone turnover resulting from secondary hyperparathyroidism, but coexistent osteomalacia may contribute in some cases. The bladder may not be visualized because of failure to excrete tracer. Absence of the bladder helps to differentiate the bone scan in renal osteodystrophy from that in other metabolic disorders.

Osteosclerosis may occasionally be seen on radiographs of the spine in patients with renal osteodystrophy; the bone scan equivalent is linear areas of increased tracer uptake corresponding to the cortical borders of vertebrae, against a background of generalized high uptake in the spine. Sites of ectopic calcification may be recognized, and the bone scan is more sensitive than routine radiography in identifying pulmonary calcification. The bone scan is also of value in the assessment of renal transplant patients complaining of bone pain. These patients may develop avascular necrosis, which is usually related to corticosteroid therapy, and involved sites are most often seen on the scan as focal areas of increased tracer uptake due to the healing osteoblastic response by surrounding bone, although in early disease photon deficient lesions may be present and are increasingly being identified in later disease with the use of SPECT (See Chapter 6).

Primary hyperparathyroidism

Primary hyperparathyroidism is a common disorder which is now being diagnosed with increasing frequency and at an earlier stage because of the availability of routine calcium estimations and parathyroid hormone assay. The degree of bone scan abnormality generally reflects the amount of skeletal involvement, and there is thus a wide range of scan appearances from normal to occasionally, those mimicking severe renal osteodystrophy. It should be emphasized that most patients have mild disease so that the bone scan usually appears normal and thus has no clear diagnostic role to play in the routine evaluation of patients with suspected primary hyperparathyroidism. Radiographic skeletal surveys are also normal in most cases, but specific changes such as sub-periosteal erosions can occasionally be seen. The bone scan is the more sensitive of the two investigations, and if the scan appearances are not suggestive of metabolic bone disease then radiographs will invariably be normal.

Focal abnormalities on the bone scan in primary hyperparathyroidism are uncommon but may be seen when brown tumours are present, with chondrocalcinosis, or following vertebral collapse. In addition, in rare instances when a patient presents with aggressive, rapidly advancing primary hyperparathyroidism, multiple sites of ectopic calcification may be seen (Fig. 4.4 A, B).

Osteomalacia

The bone scan appearances in osteomalacia are usually abnormal and will often suggest the presence of metabolic bone disease. While focal areas of increased tracer uptake cannot be considered to be metabolic features, their presence, when the scan appears characteristic of metabolic bone disease, is suggestive of pseudofractures (Fig. 4.5 A, B). The bone scan provides a sensitive means of identifying pseudofractures, particularly in the ribs, and may detect lesions which are not visualized with conventional

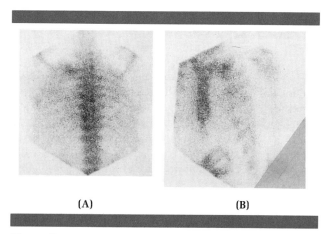

(A)   (B)

Fig. 4.4 **Bone scan views (A) posterior thoracic spine and (B) left anterior chest. There is increased tracer uptake diffusely throughout the lung fields and in addition there is tracer uptake in the left hypochondrium. This patient had hypercalcaemia and scan appearances are due to microcalcification in the lungs and stomach. It should be noted that such findings are only seen with extremely high levels of serum calcium.**

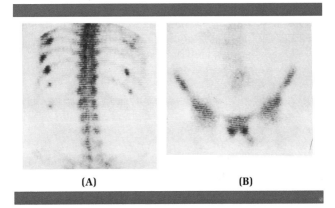

(A)   (B)

Fig. 4.5 **Bone scan views (A) posterior spine and (B) anterior pelvis. This is a case of osteomalacia with pseudo-fractures present in the ribs and both inferior pubic rami. Note the renal images are not visualized.**

radiology. However, lesions in the pelvis can on occasion be missed because of their symmetrical nature, or if they are obscured by bladder activity.

Recently, the entity of aluminium-induced osteomalacia has been recognized in uraemic patients on haemodialysis. Osteomalacia occurs because aluminium is deposited at the calcification front and blocks mineralization. Aluminium essentially acts as a bone 'poison', which is quite different from the vitamin D deficiency state normally found in osteomalacia. Scan images in this condition are of very poor quality with high background activity resulting from the relative failure of tracer to be taken up by bone. The quality of the scan images is dramatically improved following treatment with desferrioxamine.

Osteoporosis

Osteoporosis is currently an extremely topical disease as the magnitude of the related problems in terms of morbidity, mortality and indeed financial cost have become widely recognized. While the bone scan has a limited role to play in the initial diagnosis it nevertheless, has a valuable role to play in the evaluation and management of patients with osteoporosis.

Osteoporotic bones are abnormally brittle and fractures may occur. These are easily recognizable on the bone scan and are seen as focal areas of increased tracer uptake. If vertebral collapse is present, scan appearances are characteristic with an intense linear increase in tracer uptake corresponding to the site or sites of fracture (Figs. 4.6–4.8 A, B, C). This intense uptake usually fades over a period of six months to two years following collapse and thus the scan is of value in assessing the age of the vertebral collapse. In the situation of a patient known to have osteoporosis and vertebral collapse who presents with back pain, the scan may be helpful in evaluating symptomatology. Rib fractures are common in osteoporotic subjects and are easily seen on the bone scan. A normal scan would ex-

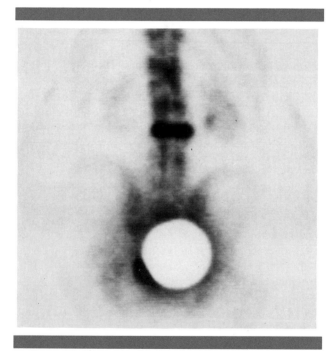

Fig. 4.6 **Posterior view of lumbar spine. There is intense linearly increased tracer uptake throughout L3 due to recent vertebral collapse.**

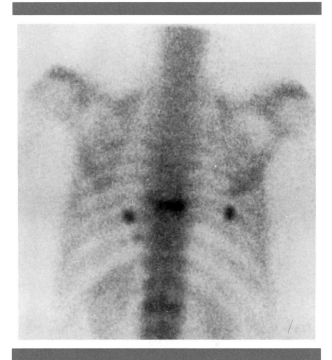

Fig. 4.7 **Posterior view of thoracic spine showing linearly increased tracer uptake in T9 and to a lesser extent in L1. Scan appearances are due to previous vertebral fractures at different stages of resolution. Note also rib fractures which are a common finding in patients with osteoporosis.**

clude recent fracture, and other causes for pain should then be considered.

The bone scan has also been used to evaluate patient symptoms while receiving sodium fluoride, a drug which stimulates osteoblastic activity. It is well-recognized that approximately 40–50% of patients receiving sodium fluoride will develop 'rheumatic' pains which have been attributed to new or activated degenerative joint disease. In such cases, scans often show new areas of increased tracer uptake, primarily at sites in the peripheral skeleton where trabecular bone is present, such as the metaphyses of long bones. There is some controversy as to whether these le-

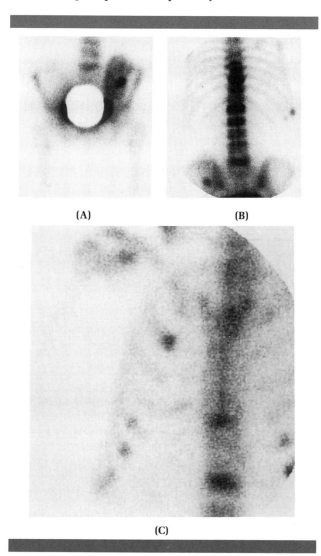

(A) (B)

(C)

Fig. 4.8 **Bone scan views (A) anterior pelvis, (B) posterior spine and (C) right anterior chest. A renal transplant patient and the functioning kidney is clearly visualized on the anterior pelvis view. This patient has severe osteoporosis due to long-term steroid therapy and multiple spinal and rib fractures are seen.**

sions reflect a periosteal reaction or are due to stress microfractures. Whatever the precise cause, it is apparent that the bone scan provides a sensitive means of monitoring the skeletal response to this drug.

Although the bone scan has a limited role to play in the dia-gnosis of osteoporosis, it may nevertheless provide valuable information in osteoporotic subjects (Table 4.1). When patients present with severe back pain and vertebral collapse, it may not always be apparent that osteoporosis is the cause and one may be concerned as to the possibility of coexistent disease, such as metastases or infection. In this situation the bone scan provides the most sensitive means of evaluating the skeleton.

Table 4.1 **Role of the bone scan in osteoporosis**

1	Baseline study for future comparison
2	Identify coexistent disease
3	Identify sites of fracture
4	Correlate fractures with clinical symptoms
5	Assess the time interval since vertebral fracture occurred

Paget's disease

Paget's disease of bone is a common disorder with an approximate incidence of 5% over the age of 55, the incidence rising with age. The disease is often asymptomatic and is discovered as an incidental finding on radiographic skeletal surveys or bone scans, or as a result of finding an elevated serum alkaline phosphatase. In recent years effective therapy (the bisphosphonates) have been introduced and it may often be appropriate to treat such cases particularly when dealing with a younger individual or if disease is extensive. In a minority of cases there is a high associated morbidity most often due to bone pain, deformity and fracture and occasionally mortality when sarcomatous change occurs. Paget's disease is usually polyostotic, but maybe monostotic in approximately 20% of cases.

Sites of bone which are affected by Paget's disease show

Bone scanning and photon absorptiometry in metabolic disease:

both a striking increase in skeletal metabolism and an increase in vascularity and there is thus high avidity for bone-seeking radiopharmaceuticals. The amount of tracer uptake in bone appears to be directly related to the degree of activity of the disease process. It has been clearly shown that the bone scan is more sensitive than routine X-ray for the detection of lesions. Further, the bone scan appearances in Paget's disease are often characteristic (Table 4.2) with the predominant feature being markedly increased uptake of tracer, which is usually distributed evenly throughout most or all of the affected bone (Figs. 4.9–4.13). A common exception to this general rule is seen in osteoporosis circumscripta (lytic disease involving the skull), where tracer uptake is most intense at the margins of the lesion.

Table 4.2 **Bone scan findings in Paget's disease**

1	Intense uptake of tracer
2	Diffuse involvement of bone
3	Anatomical features may be emphasised, eg the transverse processes in spine
4	Disease extends to the ends of long bones, rather than primarily affecting the diaphysis
5	Expansion of bone
6	Deformity of bone
7	Gradual change only over years
8	Polyostotic disease usually present
9	Spine and pelvis are the most commonly involved sites

The appearance of lesions on the bone scan are often striking and pagetic bone seems to be 'picked out' as the borders between normal and abnormal bone are well delineated. When the appendicular skeleton is involved lesions generally commence at the articular end of the bone and progress into the shaft. While the bone scan in general is sensitive for lesion detection, appearances may be non-

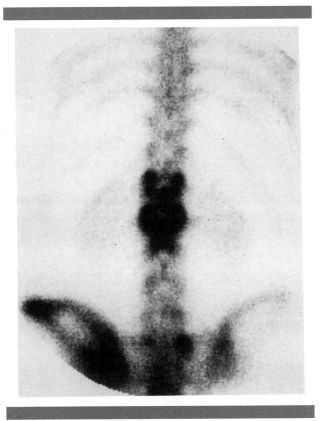

Fig. 4.9 **Posterior view of spine showing intense increased tracer uptake throughout L1 and L2 and left hemipelvis. These appearances are typically those of Paget's disease.**

specific. Nevertheless, in Paget's disease there is seldom any doubt as to the correct diagnosis, particularly when polyostotic disease is present. In doubtful cases confirmation by radiology or bone biopsy may be required.

The main advantages of the bone scan over X-ray in an individual with suspected Paget's disease are:

1. Increased sensitivity
2. Visualization of the whole skeleton

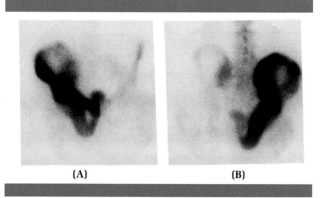

Fig. 4.10 Views of (A) anterior and (B) posterior pelvis. There is striking increased tracer uptake throughout right hemipelvis. Appearances are classically those of Paget's disease.

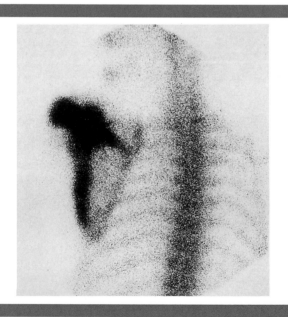

Fig. 4.11 Posterior view of thoracic spine showing intense uptake of tracer in left scapula. This is a common site for pagetic involvement.

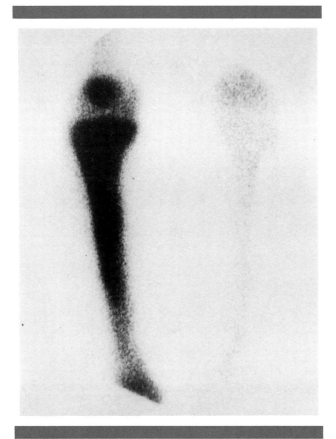

Fig. 4.12 **Anterior view of tibia showing marked increased uptake of tracer in right tibia and patella due to Paget's disease.**

3. Ease of lesion detection in 'difficult' sites such as ribs and sternum
4. Rapid evaluation of the study

It should be recognized however that it may be difficult to diagnose a fracture in pagetic bone as differentiation of a focal increase in tracer uptake from high background activity may not always be possible. This may be a particu-

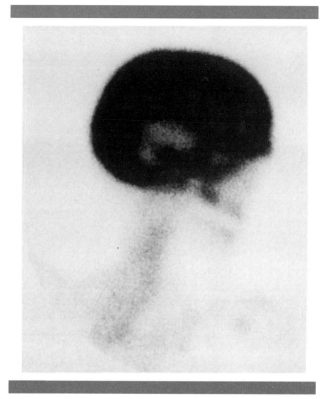

Fig. 4.13 **Lateral view of skull showing intense uptake of tracer due to Paget's disease.**

lar problem when stress fractures are present. Similarly, if sarcomatous change develops it may not be apparent on the scan, although one would be concerned about this possibility if expansion of a lesion outside normal anatomical borders occurs. If an individual has an unexpected exacerbation of symptoms or has persistent pain, fracture or sarcomatous change should be suspected and X-ray is required for further evaluation.

BONE MASS MEASUREMENTS
While many factors contribute to an individual's risk of developing osteoporosis and subsequent fracture, all seem

to act by reducing the absolute amount of bone present. Several studies have shown a clear relationship between bone strength and bone mineral content and there has therefore been considerable interest in the measurement of bone mass to assess risk of fracture.

A variety of non-invasive techniques is available for the assessment and measurement of bone mass. Some of these, for example radiographic photodensitometry, are well established, but have significant methodological problems which result in poor measurement precision. Others, such as neutron activation analysis, have been performed in research centres for some years, but are unlikely to be widely used because of their high cost and technical complexity. In the past decade, however, there have been significant advances in technologies that make accurate bone mass measurements routinely available for patient diagnosis and management. Quantitative computed tomography is one technique which has been developed for spinal bone mass measurement. It has the advantage that it can provide a measure of trabecular bone only, in regions within the vertebral cortical shell. Trabecular bone is metabolically more active than cortical bone and thus more susceptible to change. However, the technique is no more sensitive than photon absorptiometry, is more expensive in capital terms, and delivers radiation doses to the bone marrow which may be greater by a factor of the order of 100. Hence, it is unsuitable for serial studies.

Photon absorptiometry

The most widely used techniques for bone mineral measurement are single and dual photon absorptiometry. In these systems, a highly collimated beam of low-energy photons obtained from an isotope source is directed through the tissues, and the transmitted beam intensity is monitored with a well collimated scintillation detection system. The source and detector move synchronously along a rectilinear path, over the site of interest. The measured transmission at each point is related to the quantity of bone mineral in the beam path. The techniques are calibrated by measurements on ashed bone, or solutions that are radiologically equivalent to hydroxyapatite.

Single photon absorptiometry (SPA) An iodine-125 source, emitting 28 keV X-rays, is used to provide transmission measurements through the tissues of the selected site. In the case of SPA this is almost always the distal radius. Low photon energies are used to provide maximum contrast between bone and soft tissue, although the high attenuation produced by all materials at these energies effectively limits the use of this technique to the appendicular skeleton. As variation in soft tissue thickness alone would produce transmitted beam intensity variations, the total thickness of tissue transversed by the beam must be standardized. This is achieved by surrounding the measurement site (forearm) with water or a tissue-equivalent gel, so that the only remaining variable at each measurement point is the bone mass present in the beam path. Given that the attenuation of the beam within the bone is exponential, bone mass can be computed.

Dual photon absorptiometry (DPA) In DPA, the radiation beam consists of two distinct photon energies, usually derived from a single radionuclide source. Simultaneous transmission measurements are made at two energies and thicknesses of soft tissue, and mass of bone mineral present in the beam path can then be computed. Bone density can thus be measured independently of the amount of soft tissue, and for DPA it is not necessary to ensure equal soft tissue thickness at all measurement points by immersion. In principle, all body sites can be investigated directly, including those of most clinical relevance, ie the spine and femoral neck. Commercial systems incorporate [153]Gd as the radiation source. The emitted energy spectrum has peaks around 44 keV and 100 keV, the lower energy providing good bone-to-soft tissue contrast. Scanner motion and data collection/processing are controlled by a microcomputer. Regions of interest within the scanned tissue volume can then be defined as required for assessment. In the case of the lumbar spine, bone mineral content and bone mineral per unit area in the L2 to L4 region are most commonly studied. The technique, however, cannot differentiate calcium in bone from other sources (eg degenerative disease involving the spine or aortic calcification), and such factors should be borne in mind, particularly when studying elderly subjects.

Dual energy X-ray absorptiometry
This is the latest development in absorptiometry and uses an X-ray tube rather than an isotope source for its photon flux. The dual energy peaks are obtained by either switching kilovoltage or by filtering X-rays from an X-ray generator of high stability. With the high count rate obtained scan times are speeded up considerably – a spine or femur can be measured in approximately 6 minutes. The precision is excellent and in clinical practice values in the range 0.5 – 1.2% can be achieved. Long term precision has not yet been evaluated but the technique shows considerable promise. Further advantages are that the stability of the X-ray source eliminates any errors that may arise from declining activity with an isotope source, and there is much improved resolution of images.

CLINICAL APPLICATIONS OF PHOTON ABSORPTIOMETRY

The most clinically relevant fractures are those of the spine and femoral neck, and it would therefore appear logical to measure bone mineral at these sites using DPA. It has, however, been suggested that because of higher precision, SPA measurements of the forearm constitute a more appropriate method of assessing skeletal mass in group study. It would appear, however, that while there is reasonable correlation between the forearm and the spine in normal subjects ($r = 0.7$), in disease states the correlation is much poorer. Further, in some diseases, and in particular where there is accelerated bone loss, preferential loss may occur from trabecular bone as compared to cortical bone. In addition, it has been shown that SPA is extremely poor at differentiating between osteoporotic and normal subjects, and while there is still some overlap with DPA, the separation between groups is much improved.

DPA measurements of the spine do, indeed, allow reasonable separation between osteoporotic individuals and control subjects, and it has even been suggested that a fracture threshold can now be defined, below which individuals are at high risk of sustaining a fracture. While studies have shown a good correlation between vertebral fracture and bone mineral content of the spine, other studies have shown only a weak correlation between femoral neck fractures and bone mineral. This may be particularly important, as fracture of the femur is of much greater clinical and, indeed, economic, relevance than fracture of the spine.

Bone mineral measurements, however, need not be used routinely in the evaluation of patients with established osteoporosis as results will, inevitably, be low and, indeed, anyone over the age of 75 years will have low values. Such measurements may, however, be important in an osteoporotic individual to assess the response to therapy such as fluoride. The main routine application of bone mineral measurements is in the younger individual to assess how good or otherwise skeletal mass is, eg a woman who is in her early post-menopausal years and who has a strong family history of osteoporosis, but is reluctant to take long-term hormonal replacement therapy unless this is absolutely necessary. The greatest potential role for bone mass measurements is in screening the normal population to assess risk of subsequent osteoporosis. Clearly this is still a contentious issue, but in view of the magnitude of the problem with regard to patient morbidity and financial cost, some co-ordinated approach to prevention of bone loss will eventually have to be instigated. In general, risk factors such as a woman being blonde, thin or a smoker are crude in terms of assessment of whether a woman will develop osteoporosis. If screening programmes are to be introduced then much more precise information would be required to deal with the many millions of women involved. Bone mass measurements provide the single best assessment of subsequent risk of fracture.

Fractures remain the most common bone lesion. These are usually apparent from the clinical evidence and X-rays are clearly the initial diagnostic technique. It is nevertheless important to be familiar with the scan appearances of fracture as these, for example in ribs, are commonly seen as incidental findings (Figs. 5.1A, B–5.2) and should be correctly interpreted. There are, however, many situations when X-rays will initially fail to diagnose an injury and indeed it is not uncommon for patients with stress fractures to have a normal X-ray when they first become symptomatic. Also, some injuries may not be diagnosed by X-ray but can be detected easily by bone scan, eg shin

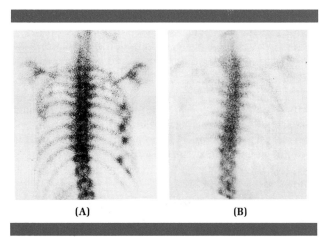

(A)   (B)

Fig. 5.1 **Bone scans, (A) Posterior thoracic spine, (B) Nine months later. On the original image there are multiple focal lesions in the right posterior ribs which are linear. These are the typical appearances of benign fracture. On the subsequent image there has been resolution of disease.**

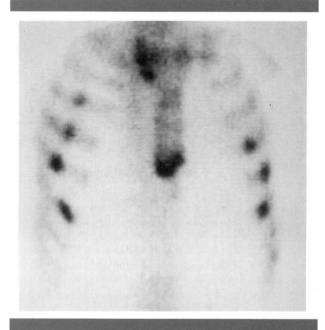

Fig. 5.2 **Anterior view of thorax. Multiple lesions are present in the ribs in a linear pattern and in the lower sternum. Appearances are due to fractures in the ribs and sternum following successful and enthusiastic cardiac resuscitation.**

splints. As the public becomes more aware of physical health, there is increasing participation in all forms of sport and correspondingly a rising incidence of sports-related bone and soft tissue injury.

OCCULT FRACTURE

While the great majority of fractures will be detected by standard X-ray techniques, on occasion this will not initially reveal a suspected fracture, eg scaphoid (Fig. 5.3) or ribs, or less commonly neck of femur. However, confirmation of fracture will usually be found on a later, repeat X-ray examination. The bone scan may also provide diagnostic information in a symptomatic individual with an X-ray

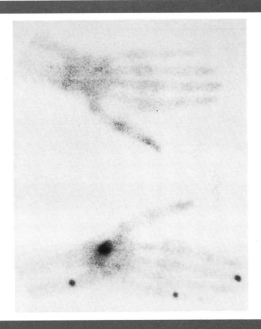

Fig. 5.3 **View of hands. There is an intense focal lesion in the left scaphoid. The clinical history would suggest a fracture but the initial X-ray was negative, although a subsequent study confirmed the scan diagnosis of fracture.**

finding which may be of clinical relevance but could be due to a congenital abnormality, eg is there a bipartate sesamoid bone or a recent fracture (Fig. 5.4 A, B, C)? On occasion the bone scan may clarify the cause of persistent pain following fracture, eg due to Sudeck's atrophy (Fig. 5.5). The sensitivity of bone scanning may be further enhanced with SPECT studies (Fig. 5.6 A – E).

It is now recognized that the bone scan will identify a fracture within 24 hours of injury in 95% of cases under 65 years of age. In older patients the detection of fracture may be delayed by 48 to 72 hours. A false negative study can also rarely be obtained in patients taking high doses of steroids. However, in general all fractures will be detected

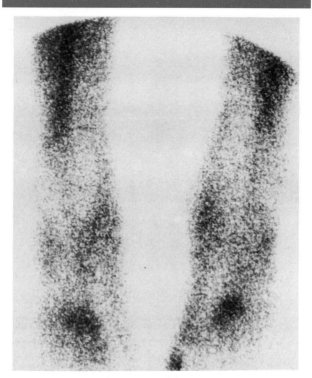

Fig. 5.4 (A)

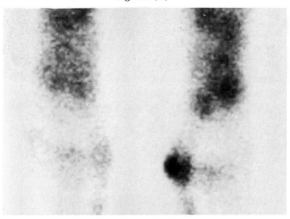

Fig. 5.4 (B)

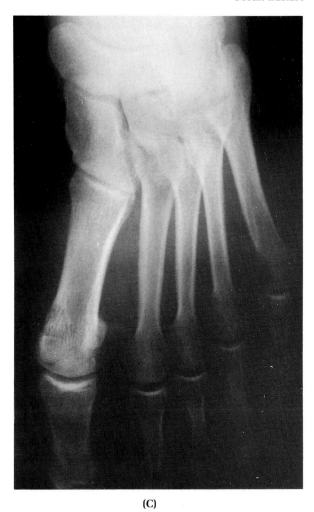

(C)

Fig. 5.4 Bone scan views of feet. (A) Blood pool, (B) Delayed image and (C) X-ray of left foot. This patient complained of pain in the left big toe. X-ray (C) revealed a bipartate sesamoid bone. While this was the site of the patient's pain it was not apparent whether the radiological abnormality was congenital or due to fracture. The bone scan clearly shows increased vascularity and metabolic activity at this site confirming fracture.

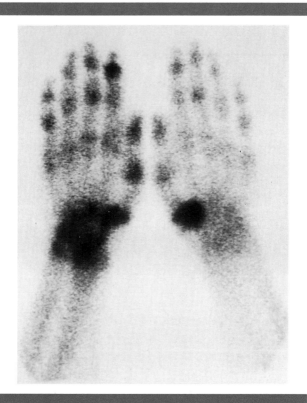

Fig. 5.5 This 67-year-old woman sustained a right-sided Colles'
fracture five months previously but continued to complain of
pain in her wrist. Bone scan of hands shows increased tracer
uptake in the distal right radius at the site of known fracture.
There is also extensive severe osteoarthritis involving many
small joints in the fingers and both first metacarpal/carpal
joints. Note, however, that there is diffusely increased tracer
uptake in the right forearm, wrist and hand when compared
with the left. This finding is typical of Sudeck's atrophy.

on the bone scan by 72 hours after injury and conversely,
a negative bone scan at 72 hours excludes significant bone
injury.

It should be noted that the time interval following fracture for the bone scan appearances to return to normal is

considerably longer than the time for clinical or even X-ray healing. This is explained by the fact that the scan reflects the osteoblastic response, and increased metabolic activity at the fracture site continues for a significant period following clinical improvement. The bone scan appearances generally resolve by 6–9 months after injury but compound fractures and fractures which are reduced during surgery or treated with orthopaedic devices may require a considerably longer time for the bone scan to return to normal. In addition patients with delayed union or non-

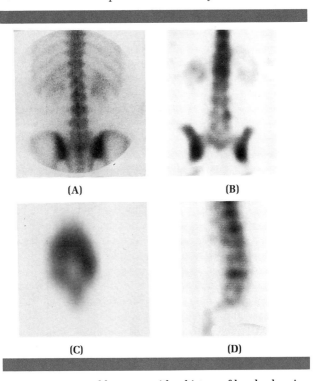

(A)   (B)

(C)   (D)

Fig. 5.6 **A 30-year-old woman with a history of low back pain. X-ray of spine suggested slight sclerosis of the left pedicle of L4. Bone scan views of the lumbar spine (A) planar and SPECT, (B) coronal, (C) transaxial, (D) sagittal. The planar image of the lumbar spine is normal but on SPECT images there is focal increased tracer uptake present in the region of the left pedicle of L4.**

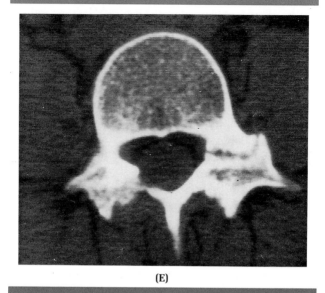

(E)

Fig. 5.6 **(E) CT of L4. CT reveals appearances compatible with previous fracture at this site.**

union may show prolonged abnormalities on the bone scan. It is important to be aware of a past history of trauma when scanning for suspected metastases, as such lesions may be incorrectly interpreted. However, prolonged persistence of bone scan abnormalities following fracture is unusual unless there was poor alignment of fracture or secondary development of degenerative disease.

In general the bone scan has not been found to provide reliable information in predicting non-union and is therefore of limited use in this situation. The bone scan however, will confirm that bone is viable and such information can be of value.

STRESS FRACTURE

Stress fractures usually arise from repeated stresses to a bone, with a resultant injury where the skeletal reparative processes are unable to cope with the damage. Such injuries are often seen in athletes with excessively heavy training regimes or else in untrained individuals or military recruits who participate in new types of exercise. X-rays may be of limited value in detecting the acute stress fracture as radiographic changes are often delayed. Early diagnosis is of practical relevance as a stress fracture of the tibia will require immobilization for approximately six weeks. If such an individual continues to exercise then there is significant risk of complete fracture. Thus in recent years the diagnosis of such abnormalities has become dependent primarily on nuclear medicine techniques. It should be recognized however, that on the bone scan images there is a spectrum of abnormality that may be seen ranging from slight increased tracer uptake running along the cortical border of a bone and reflecting periosteal injury, to an intense focus of increased tracer uptake extending throughout the entire cortex and representing true stress fracture (Figs. 5.7–5.10). It is apparent that accurate diagnosis requires at least two views of the affected bone, for example a lesion may appear to be a focal abnormality on an anterior view and yet be seen to be superficial on a lateral view. As previously stated, the specific type of abnormality will affect the clinical management. A true stress fracture requires at least six weeks rest whereas a lesser abnormality may require only a week or two of rest. It is probable that the lesser periosteal abnormalities will never show an abnormality on the radiograph, while the more prominent lesions will show changes on X-ray after a week or so.

SHIN SPLINTS

Shin splints is an important differential diagnosis of pain in a lower limb in a physically active individual. Typically the pain is in the posterior medial aspect of the tibia and is due to a periosteal reaction at the site of insertion of the tibialis posterior and soleus muscle groups. On the bone scan increased tracer uptake is seen running along the cortical border of the posterior aspect of the lower third of the tibia (Figs. 5.9 A–D, 5.10 A, B). It should be noted that this appearance will not be identified if anterior views only are obtained and if an abnormality is found without lateral views it will be considered to be a focal defect due to a stress fracture. On the lateral view the diagnosis should become apparent. Patients with shin splints are not at risk of fracture and only require to rest to avoid further pain. Light exercise is acceptable within the realms of comfort.

NON-ACCIDENTAL INJURY OF CHILDHOOD

Most often when non-accidental injury of childhood is suspected, a radiological skeletal survey is obtained which may confirm the diagnosis, particularly when metaphyseal lesions are present. However, the bone scan may be useful when an equivocal lesion is identified on X-ray and the bone scan reveals multiple lesions throughout the skeleton (Figs. 5.11–5.12). Certainly the bone scan is supe-

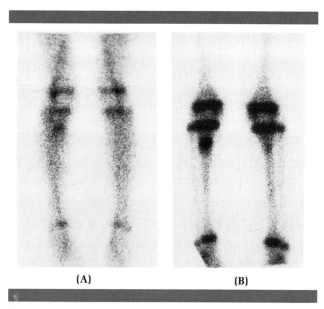

(A) **(B)**

Fig. 5.7 **A 10-year-old girl with a pain in her right upper leg. Bone scan view of tibiae, (A) blood pool and (B) delayed image. There is a vascular, metabolically active lesion present in the right upper tibia in keeping with a stress fracture. Initial X-rays were negative and although there was no clear history of trauma, subsequent X-ray revealed a sclerotic line at this site confirming the diagnosis of a stress fracture.**

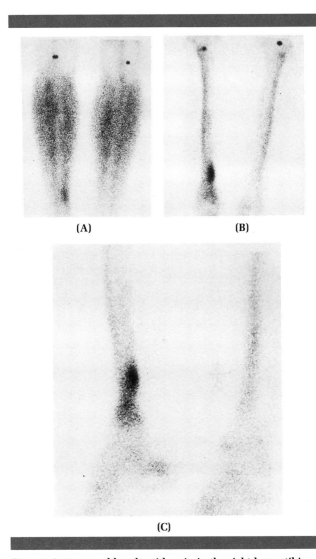

(A)

(B)

(C)

Fig. 5.8 **A 24-year-old male with pain in the right lower tibia.**
Bone scan views of tibiae (A) blood pool and delayed image,
(B) anterior and (C) lateral view. There is an intense focal area
of increased tracer uptake in the mediae aspect of right lower
tibia. The lesion is vascular and the scan appearances are in
keeping with a stress fracture.

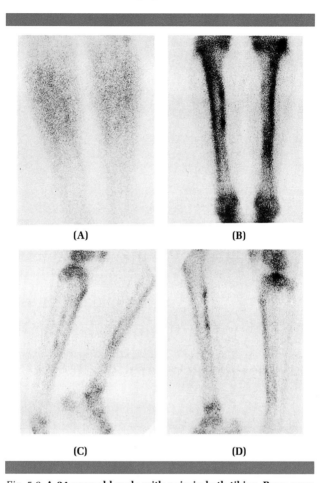

(A)

(B)

(C)

(D)

Fig. 5.9 A **24-year-old male with pain in both tibiae.** Bone scan views of tibiae (A) blood pool, delayed, (B) anterior, (C) right lateral and (D) left lateral. While on the anterior view of the tibiae there is a suggestion of focal disease particularly in the right tibiae, on the lateral view it is apparent that there is increased uptake running along the cortical aspects, particularly posteriorly. These are the appearance of shin-splints. Note that there is no significant increase in vascularity to the tibiae.

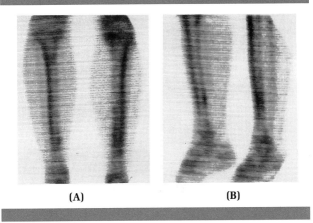

(A)   **(B)**

Fig. 5.10 A **37-year-old man with pain in the right tibia. Bone scan views of tibiae, (A) anterior and (B) left lateral. There is increased tracer uptake in the tibiae associated with the cortices. In addition there is a more focal area of increased uptake in the lower right tibia posteriorly, although this is extending along the cortical border. Appearances are most probably due to cortical hypertrophy and shin-splints. This study is nevertheless somewhat intermediate between shin-splints and stress fracture. The vascular study was negative.**

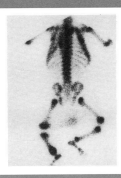

Fig. 5.11 **Bone scan view of posterior skeleton. There are multiple focal lesions present in the ribs and left lower tibia. Findings were due to non-accidental injury of childhood with multiple fractures. (Image provided by Dr H Carty.)**

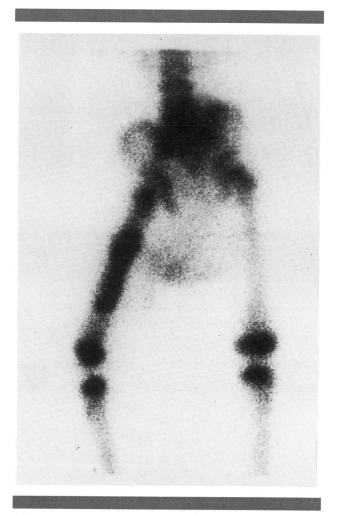

Fig. 5.12 **A further case of non-accidental injury of childhood showing a spiral fracture of the left femur.**

rior in identifying lesions in the ribs. It has been suggested that a radionuclide skeletal survey may be appropriate as the initial screening investigation and in such cases a skull X-ray should always be obtained as a skull fracture may on occasion be missed on the scan. Further it should be noted that particular care must be taken with the scanning technique as even slight patient movement will degrade the quality of the scan images. This is of particular relevance, as in children there is prominent uptake of tracer at the epiphyses—a site where fractures commonly occur. Sometimes pinhole views of the epiphyses will be of value in clarifying a possible lesion.

6 | Arthritis and Avascular Necrosis

The bone scan is of established value in the diagnosis of avascular necrosis, but has a limited role to play in the management of patients with the various arthritides. For the purpose of bone scan imaging the arthritides can be grouped into primarily inflammatory and non-inflammatory types. The classic inflammatory joint disease is rheumatoid arthritis and also included would be psoriatic and gouty arthritis, and ankylosing spondylitis. Osteoarthritis is considered a non-inflammatory condition, but as will be mentioned later, there is often a clear inflammatory component. Historically three approaches have been used with radioisotopes in the evaluation of patients with arthritis:

1. Vascular compartment markers, eg ^{131} albumin, or ^{99m}Tc-DTPA which enable visualization of the enlarged synovial blood pool when synovitis is present.
2. Inflammatory site markers, eg ^{67}Ga citrate. ^{67}Ga will concentrate in both septic and non-septic inflammatory sites and therefore has the capability to visualize the inflamed synovium directly.
3. Standard bone-seekers, formerly ^{85}Sr, ^{87}Sr and currently ^{99m}Tc diphosphonate.

In practice the last is the only approach that is currently used and indeed the standard radionuclide bone scan when performed with a dynamic and blood pool image (three phase bone scan) provides information regarding inflammation in addition to identifying any focal pathology that is present.

On the normal bone scan there is some increase of tracer uptake seen immediately adjacent to joints and in general this appears symmetrical. Therefore for a joint to appear positive on the bone scan there has to be increased tracer uptake relative to an uninvolved joint or else markedly higher tracer uptake when compared with adjacent non-articular bone.

RHEUMATOID ARTHRITIS

Inflammatory synovitis is associated with increased blood flow to the synovium and periarticular bones, and as hyperaemia is recognized as a cause of increased tracer uptake, it is likely that this is an important contributory factor to a positive bone scan in rheumatoid arthritis (Figs. 6.1 A–D, 6.2). However, the intensity of uptake of a bone-

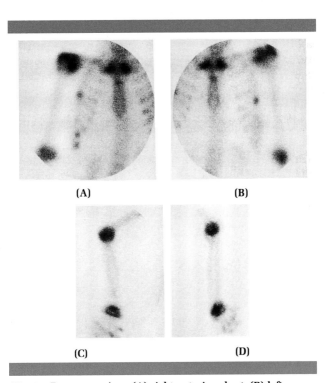

(A)   (B)

(C)   (D)

Fig. 6.1 **Bone scan views (A) right anterior chest, (B) left anterior chest, (C) right forearm, and (D) left forearm. There is increased tracer uptake present in both shoulders, elbows, wrists and hands due to rheumatoid arthritis. The rib lesions are due to fractures. The hips were not significantly involved and the patient had previous bilateral knee replacements.**

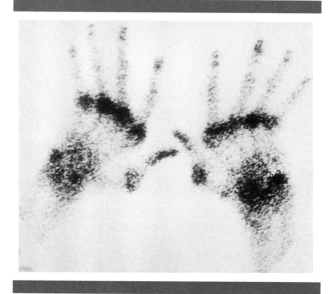

Fig. 6.2 **Bone scan view of hands. There is increased tracer uptake in many small joints of the hand and wrists in keeping with known rheumatoid arthritis. Note the ulnar deviation.**

seeking radiopharmaceutical has been found to be higher than that obtained with a blood pool imaging agent suggesting that tracer uptake in this situation is not simply related to acute inflammation alone and that there is in addition increased uptake by periarticular bone most probably due to local remodelling following bone resorption. Whatever the precise mechanism there is no doubt that in rheumatoid arthritis intense increased focal tracer uptake is seen at sites of disease. However, the scan appearances are non-specific and may be found in a wide variety of conditions including psoriatic and gouty arthritis, ankylosing spondylitis, seronegative polyarthritis, hypertrophic osteoarthropathy, reflex sympathetic dystrophy syndrome and regional migratory osteoporosis. Nevertheless, the presence of symmetrical disease with peripheral joint activity greater than axial activity, uniform involvement of the wrists and proximal joints of the limbs and feet, and typical skeletal deformities would favour a diagnosis of rheumatoid arthritis.

In rheumatoid arthritis the bone scan has been found to antedate clinical and radiographic manifestations of inflammatory synovitis, but once a diagnosis has been established a scan will not provide any additional information. It has been suggested that the bone scan may provide an accurate means of monitoring an individual's response to therapy, but any advantage in clinical practice over simpler techniques remains to be established. Therefore, the role of the bone scan in the routine management of patients with rheumatoid arthritis is limited. There is a particular problem in children due to the high tracer uptake in the epiphyses, which can obscure any increased uptake in periarticular bone reflecting synovitis and local bone remodelling. The knee is an exception as increased uptake may be identified in the patella on a lateral view. Nevertheless, the bone scan has proven to be disappointing in the management of juvenile rheumatoid arthritis.

A potential role for the bone scan is in the patient who presents with a monoarthropathy to identify cliniciallly occult joint involvement (Fig. 6.3 A, B). In practice the pick-up rate is low and the bone scan is seldom requested in such cases.

As always the value of a negative bone scan should be remembered. It has been suggested that a negative scan in a patient with polyarthralgia is adequate to exclude synovitis. However, there is relatively little evidence to support this and further studies are required. Nevertheless, a normal joint survey on bone scan in a patient with polyarthralgia is likely to be strong supportive evidence against a diagnosis of inflammatory polyarthritis.

ANKYLOSING SPONDYLITIS

Sacro-iliitis will produce a positive bone scan image and it is well established that bone scanning may identify radiologically negative sacro-iliitis in its earlier stages. The problem which arises when assessing the sacro-iliac joints on the bone scan image is that in normal subjects they are usually hotter than the surrounding pelvis and sacrum and even more so in young subjects in whom sacro-iliitis is

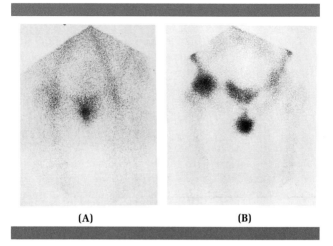

(A) (B)

Fig. 6.3 **Bone scan views of anterior pelvis, (A) blood pool and (B) delayed. There is increased tracer uptake in the right hip and there is also increased vascularity to this area. This is a 50-year-old woman with unexplained monoarthritis. There was no other abnormality on the bone scan.**

most frequently seen. While sacro-iliitis may be unilateral it is commonly bilateral and abnormality may not be apparent on subjective evaluation of the bone scan when asymmetry is not present. To overcome such difficulties various quantitative techniques have been developed whereby a ratio of count activity relating the uptake of tracer by each sacro-iliac joint to that of the body of sacrum or surrounding bone is obtained (Fig. 6.4 A, B, C). Various diagnostic indices have been proposed but individual departments who are interested in this technique need to establish their own normal range and experience as to its clinical value. Sacro-iliac joint quantitation can however, reveal abnormally high results early in the disease process when X-ray findings may be minimal or absent. Results from quantitative isotope studies tend to approach normality as end-stage fusion of the joints develops. Thus while early in the disease one may obtain a positive bone scan yet negative X-rays, in end-stage disease when metabolic activity is essentially 'burnt-out' the bone scan may be negative with marked changes identifiable on X-ray.

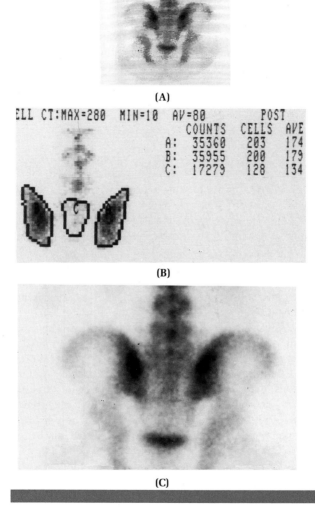

(A)

(B)

(C)

Fig. 6.4 **(A) Bone scan view of posterior pelvis. (B) Regions of interest selected over sacro-iliac joints and sacrum. (C) Sacro-iliac quantitation with index derived for each joint. This study is normal.**

In patients with ankylosing spondylitis it may be possible to identify a diffuse increase in spinal uptake of tracer most often seen in the lower dorsal spine, and in addition more focal abnormality can be seen in the apophyseal joints. As there is a tendency to bony ankylosis the scan image will often fail to clearly illustrate the normal segmental anatomy of the spine. Such appearances on the scan are of academic interest only in the presence of such dramatic radiological abnormality. However, ankylosing spondylitis may be associated with peripheral arthropathy in some 10% of cases and this can be easily identified on the radionuclide bone scan.

OSTEOARTHRITIS
In osteoarthritis increased mechanical stress occurs at altered joint surfaces and this leads to an osteoblastic reaction and reactive new bone formation which is readily demonstrated by bone scanning. Typically the scan appearances show increased tracer uptake at sites of involvement which correspond to the weight-bearing joints and distal joints of the hands and feet.

Osteoarthritis is extremely common in people over 50 years old and one must be familiar with the bone scan appearances as these will frequently be found on scans requested for a wide variety of reasons and may not be of any clinical significance. Nevertheless, the bone scan while sensitive is non-specific and in many instances further evaluation with X-ray will be necessary (Figs. 6.5–6.7). In general the degree of scan abnormality will reflect alterations in local skeletal metabolic activity and has been shown to correlate with the size of individual osteophytes. While osteoarthritis is not generally considered to be an inflammatory disease, it is apparent from three phase bone scan studies where the vascularity of lesions has been evaluated, that an inflammatory reaction is not an infrequent finding (Fig. 6.8 A, B). It may be that this simply reflects early disease where there is a significant vascular component to newly forming lesions.

Patchy tracer uptake with more focal lesions in the lower lumbar spine is a particularly common scan finding in the presence of degenerative disease. On occasion lesions may extend out from joint surfaces and will correspond to osteophytes present on X-ray. As the most common request for a bone scan is in the search for metastatic disease such appearances may occasionally lead to confusion. As stated previously it is always essential when any doubt exists to

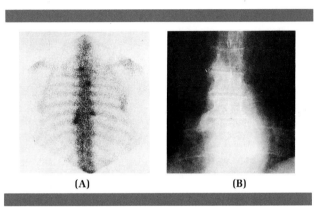

(A) (B)

Fig. 6.5 **(A) Bone scan view of posterior thoracic spine and (B) corresponding X-ray. On the bone scan there are focal areas of increased tracer uptake in upper and mid thoracic spine. These changes correspond to hypertrophic osteophyte formation on X-ray.**

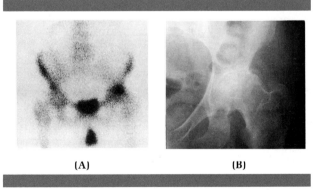

(A) (B)

Fig. 6.6 **(A) Bone scan of anterior pelvis and (B) X-ray of left hip. On the bone scan there is marked increased tracer uptake in left hip. X-ray confirms the presence of significant degenerative disease.**

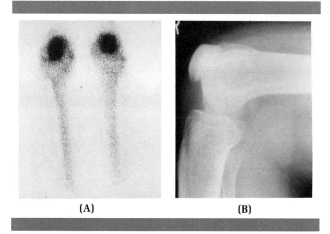

(A)   (B)

Fig. 6.7 **(A) Bone scan of tibiae. (B) Lateral X-ray of right knee. The bone scan shows increased tracer uptake in both patellae. The scan finding of 'hot' patellae is non-specific. In this case it is due to osteoarthritis of the patellofemoral joint as confirmed on X-ray (B).**

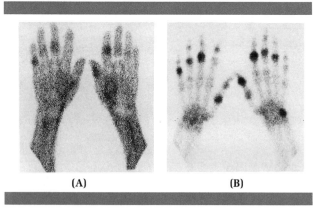

(A)   (B)

Fig. 6.8 **Bone scan of hands. (A) Blood pool and (B) delayed image. The bone scan image (B) shows the typical appearances of osteoarthritis affecting both hands. Note, however, on the blood pool image there is increased vascularity to several joints indicating an inflammatory component.**

X-ray any areas of abnormality to confirm the presence of degenerative change. In the assessment of osteoarthritis of the knee the bone scan has been shown to be more sensitive than physical examination, radiography and double contrast arthrography and it has been found that the scan provides important supplementary information in those patients in whom surgery is contemplated.

As important, and perhaps the main role of bone scanning in patients with arthritis, is to identify coexistent disease, eg tumour, infection or Paget's disease which may contribute to or indeed explain the symptoms. This is particularly relevant when symptoms are not responding as expected to therapy or the clinical course of the disease is not as predicted.

AVASCULAR NECROSIS AND BONE INFARCTION

There are a large number of disorders that may be associated with avascular necrosis and bone infarction. The more important of these include trauma, steroid therapy (Fig. 6.9), radiation, vascular injury, sickle cell disease (Fig. 6.10), Caisson disease, alcoholism with, in addition, a significant idiopathic group. The bone scan may be of considerable value in the diagnosis of avascular necrosis and is more sensitive than X-ray in this respect. MRI is however, also highly sensitive for avascular necrosis, and because of this and its superb anatomical resolution, it should be considered the imaging procedure of choice.

With avascular necrosis and bone infarction the initial pathological process in each case is bone ischaemia and scan images obtained at an early stage will show a zone of decreased tracer uptake (ie a photopenic lesion). As the pathological process continues a peripheral zone of increased tracer uptake develops which represents an osteoblastic healing response by surrounding bone. In addition, there may be secondary degenerative change. In clinical practice a hot lesion is most often seen which represents the healing response of the surrounding normal bone together with any degenerative disease that is present. While in theory a central photon-deficient area should be identifiable, this is in fact seldom seen on planar images (Fig. 6.11 A, B). With the advent of SPECT imaging this photon-deficient area can increasingly be identified and this has been found most often in the femoral head. The advantage of SPECT as stated previously, is that it is possible to study the plane of interest without any interference from surrounding structures. The femoral head is susceptible to avascular necrosis following fracture of the femoral neck and displaced fractures have a higher incidence than undisplaced ones. It has been suggested

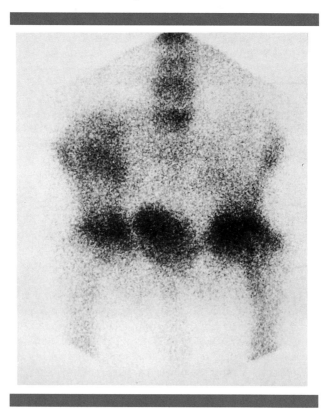

Fig. 6.9 **Bone scan view of anterior pelvis. There is increased tracer uptake in both hips due to avascular necrosis. Note the right-sided renal transplant. This patient had received high dose steroids for many years.**

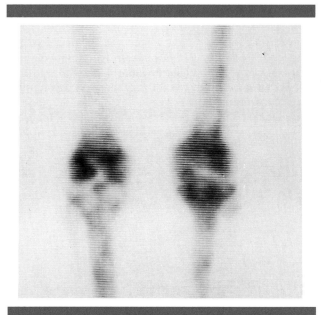

Fig. 6.10 **Bone scan view of legs. Multiple focal lesions are present due to bone infarcts in a patient with known sickle cell disease.**

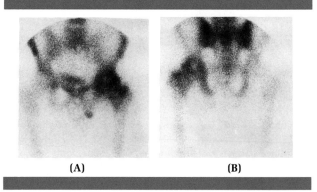

Fig. 6.11 **Bone scan views of pelvis, (A) anterior and (B) posterior. There is marked increased tracer uptake in the left hip due to avascular necrosis. This case is unusual as a central photon-deficient lesion is apparent.**

that three phase bone scanning can assist in identifying those cases with impaired vascularity and thus enable identification of those patients who may develop avascular necrosis (Fig. 6.12 A, B). However, this technique has not been proven to be reliable in clinical practice and it is seldom used as a basis for clinical decision making.

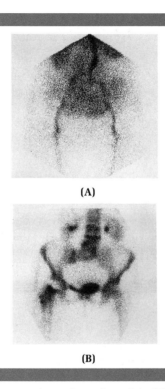

(A)

(B)

Fig. 6.12 **Bone scan views of anterior pelvis. (A) Dynamic and (B) delayed image. This patient had a right subcapital fracture of the neck of femur fixed with three screws. This study was performed two weeks later to assess the blood supply to the proximal fragment. On the delayed image there is an apparent increase in metabolic activity associated with the femoral neck and greater trochanter secondary to surgery. There is however, absent metabolic activity in the femoral head and absent blood flow to this site. These are the appearances of acute avascular necrosis of the femoral head.**

As in adults the initial indications for bone scanning in paediatrics were in patients with malignant disease. There was some reluctance to apply the technique in children with benign disease. In view of the considerable safety of bone scanning this attitude was unjustified. The great sensitivity in early pathology and the ability to obtain a whole-body skeletal image at a low radiation dose make bone scanning suitable for a variety of paediatric skeletal problems.

There are some important specific points to consider in performing a bone scan in children. It is essential to adjust the activity of ^{99m}Tc-MDP injected according to the size of the child. This is done on the basis of body surface area which can be calculated from the child's height and weight using a standard nomogram. The injected dose is then scaled down from an adult figure of 600 MBq for a standard body surface area of 1.73 m^2. In children of less than 5 kg a minimum dose of 40 MBq is employed, to ensure adequate count statistics. Injecting the tracer into very small children can be difficult and should be performed by someone who is skilled in intravenous injections in children. Prior to injection the entire procedure should be explained to the child and to the parent who should remain with the child throughout the procedure. Paediatrically trained nursing staff should be available to care for the patient. Toys and games should be provided for children who remain in the department between injection and imaging. As with adults a good fluid intake is essential following injection to aid tracer clearance and minimize the radiation dose to the bladder. In the case of children still in nappies, it should be remembered that the urine is radioactive. Precautions should be taken to reduce skin contamination with radioactive urine and arrangements made to deal appropriately with radioactive nappies.

During imaging sedation is not usually required, but sand bags fitted with wide Velcro straps can be of value in keeping the child still. All images should be obtained, if possible, with the child lying above the camera to avoid the claustrophobic feelings induced by having the camera above the patient. A modern gamma camera, with high intrinsic resolution must be used to ensure adequate visualization of skeletal detail. When imaging small structures, such as the femoral head, magnification using a converging collimator or pinhole collimator is of great value.

Bone scan abnormalities in children may be subtle and are often detected only after careful comparison with the corresponding contralateral part of the skeleton. It is essential, therefore, always to obtain high quality bone scan images of the site of suspected pathology and of the same skeletal site on the other side of the body. A good quality X-ray of the abnormal area is also essential to obtain maximum sensitivity and specificity.

The major difference in the appearance of a paediatric bone scan is the presence of the epiphyses. These growth plates are areas of major osteoblastic activity and consequently appear as areas of increased uptake on the bone scan (Fig. 7.1). It is important to recognize this appearance as normal and not due to pathology. The intense uptake in the epiphyses also may make it difficult to detect small lesions in bone adjacent to the epiphyses. If lesions are suspected close to an epiphysis, magnified views using the pinhole or converging collimator are essential.

It should also be noted that gallium-67 citrate is taken up actively in the epiphyses (Fig. 7.2). Knowledge of this appearance is of particular importance in children with suspected osteomyelitis, as normal epiphyseal uptake of ^{67}Ga should not be confused with infection.

PAEDIATRIC MALIGNANCY

The indications for bone scanning in children with malignant disease are essentially the same as in adults, that is, clinical suspicion of malignancy, staging of the extent of disease and assessing the response to therapy (see Chapter 2). The spectrum of tumours in children is of course different from adults but the skeletal response to metastatic invasion is similar – an osteoblastic reaction is produced. The typical bone scan appearance of metastases in a child is therefore of hot spots.

Haematological malignancies, particularly acute leukaemias, are among the most common paediatric tumours. Bone, as opposed to marrow, involvement is rare and bone scanning is indicated only when the child presents with bone pain or other clinical evidence of bone invasion. Similarly, in the primary CNS malignancies seen in children the bone scan is not usually required.

In children with primary malignant bone tumours a bone scan is often obtained at presentation to ensure that the

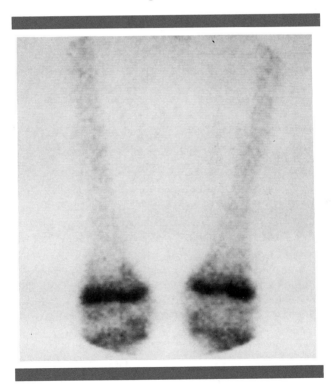

Fig. 7.1 **Bone scan of femora from 18-year-old man. Linearly increased uptake is seen in the epiphysis around the knees.**

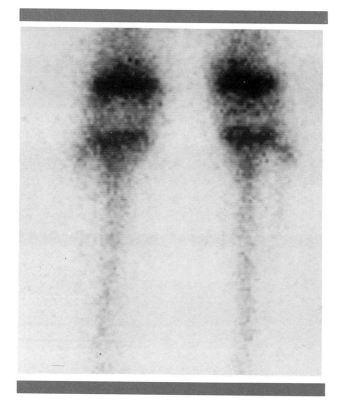

Fig. 7.2 **Gallium-67 scan of knees from 14-year-old girl.
Increased tracer uptake is seen in the (normal) epiphysis
around the knees.**

rest of the skeleton is normal (Fig. 7.3 A, B). The use of
routine bone scans during follow-up in the absence of
symptoms is controversial and most centres do not follow
this policy, but obtain studies when clinically indicated
(Fig. 7.4). It should be remembered that benign bone
tumours may produce intense uptake of bone scan agents
(Figs. 7.5, 7.6).

Neuroblastoma is a paediatric tumour which frequently
metastasises to bone, and a bone scan should be part of the
initial staging of patients with this tumour. All patients
with neuroblastoma should also be imaged using ^{132}I or ^{131}I

labelled met-iodobenzylguanidine (mIBG), which has high affinity for soft tissue and bone marrow lesions in neuroblastoma (Fig. 7.7 A, B). Bone scanning and mIBG imaging are complementary in neuroblastoma as each may demonstrate lesions missed by the other. The primary tumour may show ^{99m}Tc-diphosphonate uptake (Fig. 7.8) but this is not a reliable means of detecting soft tissue disease. Bone metastases in neuroblastoma may be subtle and present as diffusely increased uptake in the metaphysis of a limb bone.

The use of the bone scan in histiocytosis-X is controversial. Some authors believe that it is useful in demonstrating the extent of skeletal involvement by this condition, but the majority view is that it misses some lesions and an X-ray skeletal survey is preferable.

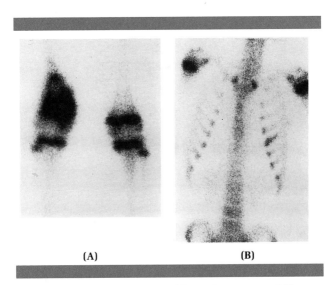

(A)   (B)

Fig. 7.3 (A) Anterior bone scan of knees from 9-year-old boy with osteosarcoma of the right lower femur. The bone scan appearances are typical. (B) Anterior views of chest shows increased uptake in the anterior end of the left 6th rib. Bone biopsy showed a metastasis. (Images courtesy of Dr JR MacKenzie.)

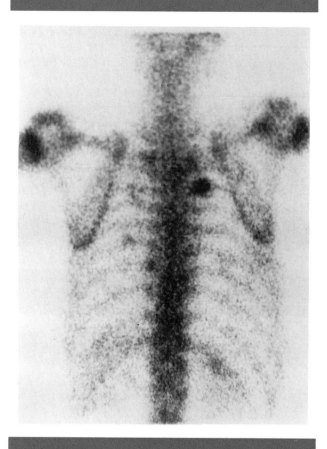

Fig. 7.4 **Posterior bone scan of chest from 13-year-old boy with osteosarcoma of left femur diagnosed three years previously. Multiple bone metastases are apparent. (Image courtesy of Dr JR MacKenzie.)**

BONE AND JOINT INFECTION IN CHILDREN

Children are particularly susceptible to osteomyelitis, which in them characteristically occurs in the metaphysis of the bone (see Chapter 3). In a child with suspected osteomyelitis the first investigation should be an X-ray of the af-

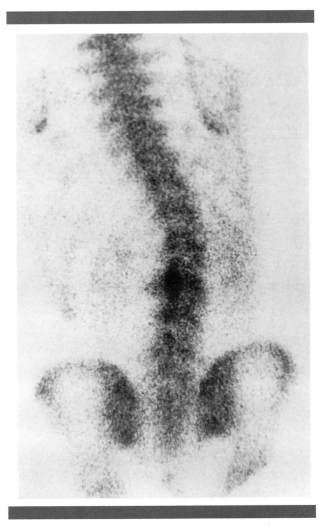

Fig. 7.5 **Posterior bone scan of lumbar spine and lower thoracic spine from a 15-year-old girl with a painful scoliosis. A focal area of increased uptake is seen in L2. X-rays showed no specific changes. Biopsy demonstrated an osteoid osteoma. (Image courtesy of Dr JR MacKenzie.)**

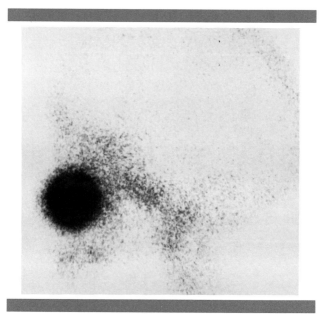

Fig. 7.6 Left lateral view of skull from a 6-year-old girl with fibrous dysplasia of the maxilla. (Image courtesy of Dr JR MacKenzie.)

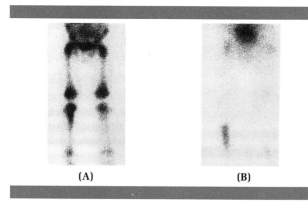

(A)   (B)

Fig. 7.7 (A) Anterior bone scan of the legs in an 18-month-old boy with neuroblastoma. There is increased uptake in the right upper tibia due to a bone metastasis. (B) Increased uptake is seen at the same site on the ^{131}I-mIBG study. (Images courtesy of Dr JR MacKenzie.)

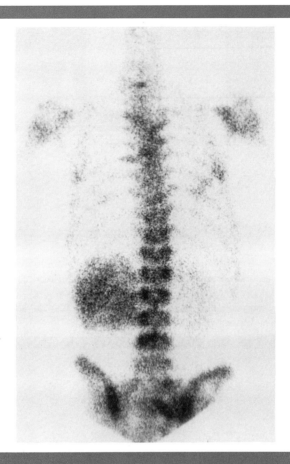

Fig. 7.8 **Posterior bone scan of spine in 12-year-old boy with a left-sided neuroblastoma. Marked uptake in the primary tumour is evident. There are also multiple bony metastases. (Image courtesy of Dr JR MacKenzie.)**

fected site. If this is negative a three phase bone scan should be obtained (Fig. 7.9 A, B). Special views may be necessary to confirm subtle or questionable abnormalities (Fig. 7.10 A, B, C). It should be remembered that the bone scan may not be positive in the first 24–48 hours after the onset of symptoms and that the first bone scan change in

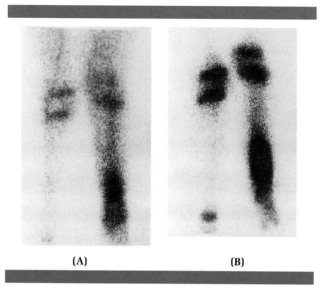

(A)   (B)

Fig. 7.9 (A) Increased uptake on the blood pool and (B) static bone images due to tibial osteomyelitis in a 10-year-old girl. (Images courtesy of Dr JR MacKenzie.)

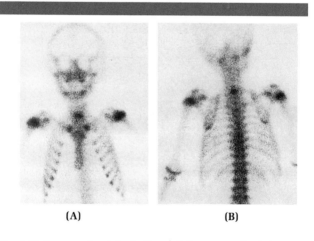

(A)   (B)

Fig. 7.10 Increased uptake in the neck is seen on the (A) anterior and (B) posterior bone scan images from an 8-year-old girl with torticollis. It is unclear whether this is in cervical spine or anterior neck.

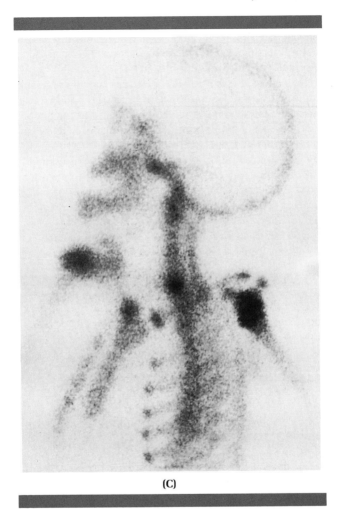

(C)

Fig. 7.10 **An oblique view (C) shows clearly the abnormality is in the cervical spine. A diagnosis of cervical spine osteomyelitis was subsequently made.**

infection may be a photopenic (cold) lesion (Fig. 7.11 A, B, C). Areas of abnormality on the bone scan should be examined with localized radiography, using special views as required. If the cause of the bone scan abnormality remains uncertain a biopsy should be obtained. In some patients with a negative bone scan a suspicion of osteomyelitis may persist. Gallium-67 or labelled leucocyte imaging can be helpful in this context, but are used sparingly because of the relatively high radiation dose.

In acute septic arthritis the bone scan may be normal in the early stages. The presence of increased uptake in the periarticular bone may indicate osteomyelitis but can also be the result of hyperaemia. The bone scan therefore has a limited role in septic arthritis which should be diagnosed by joint aspiration. In more chronic arthritis a normal X-ray the bone scan can be helpful, as the finding of a focal hot spot suggests the presence of an alternative pathology such as a Brodie's abscess, an osteoid osteoma or, rarely, malignancy.

Special problems may be encountered when osteomyelitis is suspected in a neonate. A positive bone scan is

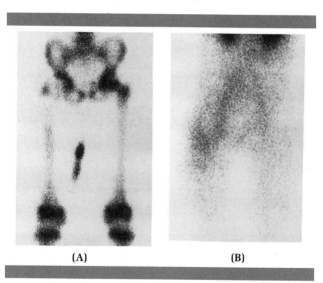

(A) (B)

Fig. 7.11 **(A) Anterior view of pelvis and femora from a 7-year-old girl with a painful right hip. There is decreased uptake in the right femoral head and upper femoral shaft due to osteomyelitis. Radioactive urine can be seen in a urinary catheter. Three weeks later a blood pool image (B) shows decreased activity in the region of the femoral head and hyperaemia in the upper thigh.**

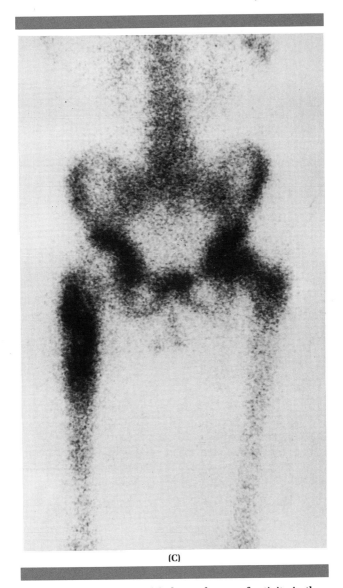

(C)

Fig. 7.11 **The static image (C) shows absence of activity in the right femoral head, reflecting bone necrosis, and increased uptake in the upper right femoral shaft. (Images courtesy Dr JR MacKenzie.)**

helpful in such a patient, but the value of a negative study is more questionable. Some series have suggested that there is a high incidence of false negative bone scans in osteomyelitis in this age group. It is possible that modern high resolution gamma cameras, use of magnification techniques and a careful search for subtle changes may improve the pick-up rate. It remains possible, however, that the neonatal skeleton shows a different response to infection and a negative bone scan in this context must be viewed with caution. Labelled white cell imaging has been reported to give positive results in some very young infants with osteomyelitis.

THE PAINFUL HIP

There are multiple causes of hip pain in children of which transient synovitis, infection, Perthes' disease and slipped femoral epiphysis are the most common. Transient synovitis will produce increased activity on the blood pool image but a normal delayed image. In Perthes' disease the bone scan will demonstrate decreased uptake in the femoral head in the early stages (Fig. 7.12 A, B, C). Decreased uptake can also be produced by other causes of avascular necrosis such as sickle cell disease, though in this condition abnormalities confined to the hip are rare. In the later stages the photopenic area is gradually replaced by increased uptake representing the bone repair. The bone scan appearances of septic arthritis, osteomyelitis and bone tumours have been discussed above.

In a child with a painful joint and normal X-rays a bone scan is of great value though it should be preceded by joint aspiration if septic arthritis is suspected.

TRAUMA

Bone trauma in children can usually be imaged satisfactorily by standard radiology. The bone scan may be of value, however, in identifying multiple sites of trauma in cases of non-accidental injury (see Chapter 5). Because of the non-specificity of the bone scan an X-ray must be obtained of each abnormal area. X-rays of the skull should always be obtained in suspected non-accidental injury as fractures in

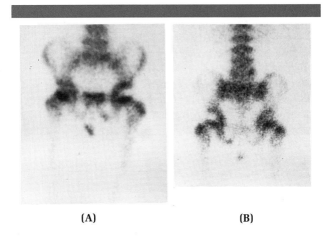

(A)   (B)

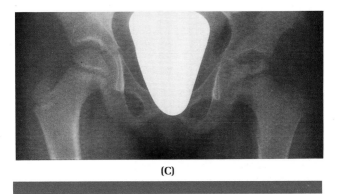

(C)

Fig. 7.12 (A) Anterior and (B) posterior bone scans of pelvis and femora from a 5-year-old girl with a painful left hip. A wedge-shaped area of decreased uptake is seen in the left femoral head indicating Perthes' disease. Bone X-rays were normal at this time but two months later (C) showed typical changes. (Images courtesy Dr JR MacKenzie.)

this site may fail to show on the bone scan. A characteristic of non-accidental injury is that there are lesions of different ages – this cannot be judged from the bone scan, but only from X-rays. For this reason and because of the non-specificity the legal status of the bone scan as evidence of non-accidental injury is uncertain at present.

As in adults the bone scan may be of value in the identification of stress fractures.

References

CHAPTER 1

Fogelman I 1987 Bone scanning in clinical practice. Springer-Verlag, London

McCook BM, Sandler MP, Powers TA, Weaver GR, Nance EP 1989 Correlative bone imaging. In: Freeman LM, Weissmann HS Nuclear Medicine Annual 1989. Raven Press, New York. pp. 143 – 177

Rosenthall L, Lisbona R 1984 Skeletal Imaging. Appleton-Century-Crofts, Norwalk Connecticut

Silberstein EB (ed) 1984 Bone Scintigraphy. Futura Publishing Company, Mount Kisco New York

CHAPTER 2

McKillop JH 1986 Radionuclide bone imaging for staging and follow-up of secondary malignancy. Clinics in Oncology **5:** 125 – 140

McNeil BJ 1984 Value of bone scanning in neoplastic disease. Seminars in Nuclear Medicine **14:** 277 – 286

Merrick MV 1989 Bone scintigraphy – an update. Clinical Radiology **40:** 231 – 232

Murray IPC, Elison BS 1986 Radionuclide bone imaging for primary bone malignancy. Clinics in Oncology **5:** 141 – 158

Robinson RG 1990 Systemic radioisotope therapy for primary and metastic bone cancer. Journal of Nuclear Medicine **31:** 1326 – 1327

CHAPTER 3

McAfee JG 1990 What is the best method for imaging focal infections? Journal of Nuclear Medicine **31:** 413 – 416

Mack JM, Spencer RP 1990 Role of radiopharmaceuticals in detection of osteomyelitis. In: Freeman LM, Weissmann HS (eds) Nuclear Medicine Annual 1990. Raven Press, New York. pp. 175 – 190

Mido K, Navarro DA, Segall GM, McDougall IR 1987 The role of bone scanning, gallium and indium imaging in infection. In: Fogelman I (ed) Bone scanning in clinical practice. Springer-Verlag, London pp. 105 – 120

CHAPTER 4

Fogelman I 1987 The bone scan in metabolic bone disease. In: Fogelman I (ed) Bone scanning in clinical practice. Springer-Verlag, London. pp. 73 – 87

Fogelman I 1990 Bone scanning in osteoporosis – the role of the bone scan and photon absorptiometry. In: Freeman LM, Weissmann HS (eds) Nuclear Medicine Annual 1990. Raven Press, New York. pp. 1 – 36

Merrick MV, Merrick JM 1985 Observations on the natural history of Paget's disease. Clinical Radiology **36:** 169 – 174

Meunier PJ, Salson C, Matthieu L, Chapuy MC, Delmas P, Alexandre C, Charhou S 1987 Skeletal distribution and biochemical parameters of Paget's disease. Clinical Orthopaedics **217:** 37 – 44

Vallenga CJLR, Pauwels EKJ, Bijvoet OLM, Frijlink WB, Mulder JD, Hermans J 1984 Untreated Paget's disease of bone studied by scintigraphy. Radiology **153:** 799 – 805

CHAPTER 5

Matin P 1988 Basic principles of nuclear medicine techniques for detection and evaluation of trauma and sports medicine injuries. Seminars in Nuclear Medicine **18:** 90 – 112

Zwas ST, Frank G 1989 The role of bone scintigraphy in stress and overuse injuries. In: Freeman LM, Weissmann HS Nuclear Medicine Annual 1989. Raven Press, New York. pp. 109 – 141

CHAPTER 6

Collier BD, Carrera GF, Johnson RP et al 1985 Detection of femoral head avascular necrosis in adults by SPECT. Journal of Nuclear Medicine **26:** 979 – 987

Rosenthall L 1987 The bone scan in arthritis. In: Fogelman

I (ed) Bone scanning in clinical practice. Springer-Verlag, London. pp. 133 – 150

CHAPTER 7
Gordon I, Peters AM 1987 The bone scan in paediatrics. In: Fogelman I (ed) Bone scanning in clinical practice. Springer-Verlag, London. 189 – 209
Murray IPC 1980 Bone scanning in the child and young adult. Skeletal Radiology **5:** 65 – 76

Index

Index

Index